WOMEN'S HEALTH QUESTIONS ANSWERED

WOMEN'S HEALTH QUESTIONS ANSWERED

A guide to over 500 common health problems

Dr PAT LAST and ANN RUSHTON

Thorsons Publishing Group

First published 1990

British Library Cataloguing in Publication Data

Last, Pat
  Women's health questions answered.
  1. Women health
  I. Title   II. Rushton, Ann
  613'.0424

ISBN 0-7225-1946-X

Published by Thorsons Publishers Limited, Wellingborough, Northamptonshire NN8 2RQ, England

Typeset by Harper Phototypesetters Limited, Northampton, England
Printed in Great Britain by Mackays of Chatham, Kent

10 9 8 7 6 5 4 3 2 1

Contents

Introduction

I qualified as a doctor from London University over 30 years ago. Women doctors were less common then. This fact, together with my specialist training in women's diseases, has ensured that over these 30 years I have responded to many thousands of questions about all aspects of health from my women patients.

My further experience as a medical journalist on the weekly magazine — *Woman's Realm* — has taught me that simple questions can cause a lot of heartache — and simple answers can give enormous help.

Questions are questions the world over and Ann Rushton and I have done our best to answer the questions that have been most commonly asked throughout the years of my practice. An invaluable aid in getting extra help is the Information Register which you will find at the back of the book. Here we have listed many organizations that offer help, counselling and advice. So if you live in the UK, Australia or the USA — or are just travelling to any of these countries — then we hope you will find this book of help to you.

Pat Last
Ann Rushton

1
How healthy are you?

Most of us only think about our health when we are ill. That's natural, but we should also value good health enough to think about it all the time. Our everyday state of health can make so much difference to how often we become ill, what ailments we suffer from and how fast we recover. There are a few simple guidelines to assess your own general health and the following questions will help you do that:

How do you weigh in?

Our weight is not static. We all fluctuate by a few pounds, or stones, depending on our age, habits and circumstances. Many women put on some weight just before a period, for example, or when giving up smoking, or going on the Pill. You want to keep within your 'ideal' weight for optimum health because to be either over- or underweight can cause problems. Being overweight can lead to heart disease, diabetes, strokes and certain forms of cancer; being underweight can also make you more susceptible to illness and — in extreme cases of undereating — can cause the periods to stop, and bring on severe vitamin and mineral deficiencies.

For a quick check on how much fat you are carrying, pinch yourself at the waist or upper arm. If you can grasp more than an inch of flesh then you need to tone up and lose some weight. To find your ideal weight against your height check the chart.

**height ft,
  in(cm)**

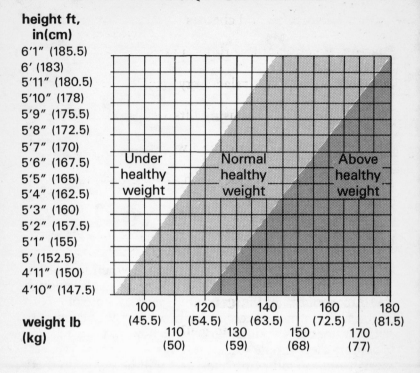

6'1" (185.5)
6' (183)
5'11" (180.5)
5'10" (178)
5'9" (175.5)
5'8" (172.5)
5'7" (170)
5'6" (167.5)
5'5" (165)
5'4" (162.5)
5'3" (160)
5'2" (157.5)
5'1" (155)
5' (152.5)
4'11" (150)
4'10" (147.5)

Under healthy weight

Normal healthy weight

Above healthy weight

**weight lb
(kg)**

100 (45.5)   120 (54.5)   140 (63.5)   160 (72.5)   180 (81.5)

110 (50)   130 (59)   150 (68)   170 (77)

Are you within the ideal weight limit for your height?
Yes/No

Positive health factors

How many of these apply to you?

Keep within a few pounds of your ideal weight
Yes/No
Eat fish at least once a week
Yes/No
Have wholemeal bread or whole cereals every day
Yes/No
Drink decaffeinated coffee or tea or herb tea
Yes/No
Use polyunsaturated margarines and cooking oils
Yes/No
Drink semi-skimmed or skimmed milk
Yes/No

Eat low-fat yoghurts and cheeses
Yes/No
Eat fruit more than three times a week
Yes/No
Eat fresh vegetables or salad every day
Yes/No
Walk upstairs instead of using lifts, escalators
Yes/No
Regular exercise, at least once a week
Yes/No
Use de-stressing techniques such as yoga/meditation/
massage
Yes/No

Here the more 'Yes' ticks the better, because you have obviously switched to healthier habits which are reflected in your diet and way of life.

Negative health factors

How many of these apply to you?

Smoke
Yes/No
Have more than two alcoholic drinks a day
Yes/No
Are not at your ideal weight
Yes/No
Eat red meat more than twice a week
Yes/No
Cook or eat meat without trimming off the fat
Yes/No
Regularly eat large quantities of cakes, biscuits
Yes/No
Regularly eat sweets, chocolates
Yes/No
Regularly eat fried food
Yes/No
Drink coffee or tea more than four times a day
Yes/No
Add salt to your food after cooking
Yes/No
Never or seldom have breakfast
Yes/No

Often have snacks in between meals
Yes/No
Use only butter or hard margarines
Yes/No
Use only full-fat milk, yoghurt and cheese
Yes/No
Always use lifts and escalators rather than walking
Yes/No
Regularly take headache/indigestion/constipation pills
Yes/No
Regularly use sleeping tablets/tranquillizers
Yes/No

All these items are negative factors in your life. Although taken individually they may not cause too much harm they can all be detrimental to your health. So, the fewer times you ticked 'Yes' then the healthier your outlook on life.

The fitness factor

To stay healthy your body needs regular exercise and that means having stamina, suppleness and strength. It can come from formal exercising in a gym or workout class, swimming, sports or just walking briskly so you get your heart pumping and oxygen circulating through your system. Regular exercise will strengthen joints and muscles and helps combat the effects of osteoporosis.

A simple step test will establish how efficient your heart and lungs are, but first you must know how to take your pulse. You can take the pulse either in your wrist, or in your neck — just below your jawbone close to your ear. Have a watch or clock with a second hand and count how many times your pulse beats over 15 seconds. Multiply that by four and that is your resting pulse rate for a minute. The table will show you what that means and only if your resting pulse rate is less than 100 beats a minute should you attempt the step test.

Resting pulse rate

Average for women

76 or under	Very Good
76-100	Good
100 or over	Not Very Good**

**If your pulse rate falls into this category, you should have it checked by your doctor.

The step test

Use a normal height stair of about eight inches. The bottom of a staircase is ideal for this. Step on and off the stair 24 times a minute continuously for three minutes. When you have finished wait for one minute and then take your pulse rate again and check with the table below. *Note* that if at any time you feel lightheaded or breathless then stop — it is not an endurance test, just to see what your level of aerobic fitness is.

Recovery pulse rate

Average for women

92 or under	Very Good
92-100	Good
101 or over	Not So Good

Using this as a guide you can keep testing your pulse rate after exercise to see what improvement you can make. The aim is to have as little difference as possible between your resting pulse rate and your recovery rate, though of course your age and general fitness will play a part in how quickly your heart can recover.

Diet and nutrition

Q **Why is it that some people eat lots and remain thin, whilst others seem to eat much less and get chubby?**

A Whoever had the answer to that would make their fortune, but there is certainly something in our inherited make-up which makes some people gain weight more easily than others, and vice versa. Various claims have been made that the characteristics of the fat in our bodies can alter the rate at which we metabolize our food, and this may be the answer.

Q **I come from a fairly well-built family. I do enjoy my food, but is my being overweight due to hereditary factors?**

A We cannot alter what we inherit from our family — only how we look on the outside. If you are overweight, it is no good blaming your genes, your knife and fork must carry the blame too.

Q **I have worked out my 'ideal' weight from charts for my height, etc but I find that very hard to achieve.**

A Your ideal weight is something that is very personal to you. As long as you know roughly what you should weigh then it is up to you where you feel comfortable.

Q **I am usually four or five pounds over my ideal weight and wonder how important that is?**

A Obviously it is better to be as near as you can to your ideal weight, but a few pounds over or under will not make any difference, as long as you are happy with it.

Q **There are so many diets on the market, how do you know which to choose?**

A The most important ingredient in any diet is willpower. After that, it is a matter of personal choice to find which diet you are happiest with. Some people like counting calories, others prefer meal replacement or a host of other new ideas that come and go.

Q **What is the best way to lose weight?**

A The only consistently successful way of losing weight, and keeping it off, is to have a sensible balanced diet and just eat less.

Q **Is it true that people who work hard need more food than those who don't do as much?**

A Yes it certainly is. Any form of hard physical work burns up the calories faster than just sitting down. So if you're a bricklayer or an athlete you will need more food to 'fuel' that activity than if you are a secretary or a student.

Q **Do men and women need the same amount of calories every day?**

A No, women need less calories than men — even when doing the same job. A male teacher for example may need 2,700 Kcal, while a woman teacher will need 500 Kcal less.

Q **Now that my husband and I are both retired we are eating less, but do we still need a different calorie intake?**

A Even in retirement men need more calories than women. Around 2,300 per day compared with just under 2,000 for a woman of the same age.

Healthcare

Q **I am never sure how to decide whether or not to call in the doctor.**

A It's quite a good exercise to imagine what you would do if there was no telephone. Is the situation serious enough for you to go out to the doctor's house and fetch him yourself? If it isn't, then it is possibly not serious enough to warrant a home visit.

Q **Is it better to wait until later in the day before calling the doctor?**

A Always call the doctor early rather than late. S/he would much rather deal with a problem at 8pm, not 3am.

Q **I particularly worry when one of the children is ill about whether to contact the doctor. I don't want to bother him unnecessarily, but I would appreciate some guidelines.**

A With children, if there is a history of reacting badly to mild infections then it is reasonable to report the illness early on. If you really are worried then don't delay in speaking to the doctor. No phrase makes their heart sink more than 'I didn't want to bother you', when faced with a desperately ill child in the middle of the night.

Q **I don't like to visit the doctor just for something trivial but is there anywhere else I can get advice?**

A If your local pharmacy displays a Green Cross in the window then that means that there is a registered pharmacist on the premises. They can suggest over the counter remedies and, if they think you need it, will refer you back to your own doctor.

Q **How is a pharmacist qualified to give advice?**

A A pharmacist's training is very similar to that of a doctor and they can provide valuable information about most aspects of health care.

Q **How do you take a temperature?**

A Before you use it, shake the thermometer downwards, with the bulb at the bottom, until it reads well below normal. Put it under the tongue and leave for one minute.

Q **What is a 'normal' temperature reading?**

A Body temperature can fluctuate during the day and it is what is normal for you that is important. However, the average is 98.4°F or 37°C.

Q **When is it best not to take a temperature?**

A Never take a temperature just after a bath, hot meal or drink, or a cigarette as it will give a falsely high reading.

Q **How do I clean the thermometer after use?**

A When you have finished wash the thermometer in cool water with some antiseptic added to it. *Never* wash a mercury thermometer in hot water as it will break.

Q **I am frightened of using a glass thermometer on my 3 year old as he could bite it. How else can I take his temperature?**

A You could use the glass thermometer in his armpit rather than his mouth, but it is better to use one of the new temperature strips which you press onto the skin. Your pharmacist should stock these.

Q **My little girl doesn't like having her temperature taken at all. Is there any other way of telling if she has a fever?**

A Very often the delicate skin on the back of your hand is all that is necessary. If she feels hotter than you, then she has a temperature.

Q **How long is it safe to keep medicines? Do they have a shelf life or can they be kept indefinitely?**

A There is certainly a shelf life for many medicines, but with tablets and pills it can be five or six years. Liquid medicines should be thrown away directly the course is finished and as a safety measure it is never wise to keep any medicine that you are no longer taking regularly.

Q **When visiting my mother recently I took some aspirin for a headache. They were very old and I've no idea how long she'd had them. How can I make sure she isn't keeping old medicines?**

A It's probably best to clear the cupboard out and start again. Write the date on the label of any over the counter medicines that she has and then you can check them periodically. That way you can tell how long she has been storing them.

Q Sometimes when I have been given a prescription I don't always remember what the doctor has said, but I don't like to ring up and bother him.

A Never be afraid to go back and check. Your doctor would far rather you did this than get the wrong information. If it is a large practice then the nurse can look up your prescription and give you the details you need.

Q I get a bit confused about which tablets I take after meals and which before. Can I find out without going back to see the doctor?

A If you are not sure about how to take your medicine — for example, whether it should be taken with food or on an empty stomach — then the pharmacist who dispensed the medicine will be able to give you all the information you need.

Q Is the bathroom the best place to keep a medicine chest?

A Traditionally the medicine chest is kept in the bathroom, but this is not the best place as many tablets and medicines deteriorate in the hot, steamy atmosphere.

Q Where is the best place to put a medicine chest?

A The ideal situation is near where you are going to need it in case of accident, and this is usually in the kitchen or living area. You should choose a cool and dry place, out of the reach of children.

Q **Is it always necessary to lock a medicine chest?**

A The cabinet should be secure, but it isn't necessary to keep it locked. If you must lock it up do make sure you, and other responsible family members, know where the key is kept.

Q **What should I keep in a medicine chest?**

A It depends a lot on your individual circumstances, but a fairly basic list would include the following: Clean scissors, some simple dressings or plasters, antiseptic cream or lotion, a *few* painkillers such as aspirin or paracetamol, an eyebath and solution, tweezers, a thermometer and a crepe bandage.

Q **I have read a lot about elderly people being affected by hypothermia in very cold weather. How can it be avoided?**

A Preventing hypothermia depends on maintaining a healthy body temperature, and that is not as easy as you may think. It is essential that elderly people have adequate heating; this means first having a warm home and then keeping a good body temperature — internally from food, and externally with warm clothing.

Q **My mother got hypothermia last winter and I was distressed because she didn't seem to realize how cold she'd let the house become.**

A Because hypothermia causes confusion, sufferers are less able to see their problem clearly and do something about it. It is essential that a responsible person keeps an eye on them to make sure that they are properly keeping warm.

Q I know that my parents worry about the cost of the central heating and I am worried that they keep turning it down to save money. How can I get them to keep the house at a healthy temperature and avoid hypothermia?

A With central heating, you can help by ensuring that the temperature controls and timing device are set so that they cannot be turned off without your help or knowledge.

Q I have an elderly neighbour and am worried about her getting hypothermia. What can I do to help?

A If she has no central heating, try to see that the living room and bedrooms are well insulated against draughts and properly heated. Make frequent visits to check that there are good food supplies and she's eating properly.

Q I live a long way from my parents and worry about how they manage during bad weather.

A If you live too far away to regularly visit your parents, then try to get a neighbour to help keep an eye on them and perhaps ring you if there are any problems. You could do the same for someone else's family who live near you.

Health at work

Q I work in a large and busy photocopying office with four other girls. A man who works in another section has told us that we could be harming our health with the levels of radiation coming from the machines. I have never heard of this before, but is he right?

A There are no known hazards from photocopying machines. There is no radiation, other than the light source which is harmless, and there are no volatile chemical fumes. The only problem can be with the static electricity that is created because of the warm, dry heat but although this can be a nuisance, it causes no harm whatsoever.

Q Our boss is a fresh air fanatic and keeps the office really cold. Can we do anything about it?

A In most countries there are Government regulations covering work place temperatures. In the UK, the minimum acceptable temperature is 61°F or 16°C. If it falls below that in the first hour of commencing work then you are justified in going home.

Q How important is it to have an even temperature when you're working?

A If your body temperature starts to fall then the blood and oxygen supplies to the brain become impaired and you will become less alert. Conversely, if it is too warm you will become sleepy and that too can affect your work performance.

Q I work in an open plan office with a lot of computer terminals. I have heard that other departments are installing ionizers but am not sure what benefit this will be?

A It is claimed that the conditions of most modern offices (particularly those high in synthetic materials and electrical and electronic equipment) drain away the negative ions from the air and can affect the health of the people who work in them. Ionizers produce a steady stream of negative ions which it is believed can help with concentration and work performance.

Q Can ionizers help with particular health conditions?

A Ionizers have also been said to help those with breathing difficulties associated with hayfever, asthma and sinusitis. However, not everyone responds positively to ionizers, many people find they have no effect on them one way or the other.

Hospitals and treatment

Q I subscribe to a private health insurance company through my work. Does the insurance company have its own doctors?

A Health insurance companies do not employ their own doctors, but they 'accredit' specialists. In general, if a doctor holds a consultant appointment at a hospital they have fulfilled the training requirements necessary. There are a few exceptions to this and your insurance company will be able to tell you what they are.

Q **If I need to see a specialist how do I go about finding one?**

A You do not need to 'find' a specialist yourself. Your personal doctor will advise you and refer you to the right consultant to deal with your problem.

Q **I would like to see a specialist for a second opinion on my doctor's diagnosis. I know who I want to see, do I need to go through my doctor or can I make an appointment direct?**

A The specialist will need to have a letter from your own doctor referring you. You should speak to your own doctor to arrange this first and you can then arrange your own appointment.

Q **I am going into hospital soon and they have asked me to bring my medicines with me. I thought these would be supplied by the hospital pharmacy, and am not sure exactly what to take with me.**

A You should take in either an empty bottle, with the drug name clearly labelled, or just one or two tablets. The hospital will want to check exactly what you are taking as they may need to adjust the dose, or change the prescription, once your condition has been assessed.

Q **I am going into hospital for the first time and am not sure what to do when I arrive.**

A On the day before, or the morning of, your admission, you should check with the ward where you are to be admitted that you are expected and there is a bed available. You will be given a time to arrive and when you get there, with a small overnight bag, a clerk will take your details for the admission record. You will then be taken to the ward and asked to change into your pyjamas or nightdress.

Q **When I have been admitted to hospital, do I get examined straight away?**

A After you have settled into the ward, you will probably have some blood taken and then there will be a visit from a junior hospital doctor. You will have to give all the details of your illness and proposed operation. The doctor will also carry out a full physical examination and this is the time you should discuss any problems or worries you have about the operation, or any of the hospital procedures.

Q **I am going to hospital shortly for an operation and I am dreading it. I am a very private person and the thought of being in a ward with strangers and having to use a bedpan is really worrying me.**

A This is something that does worry a lot of people if they are not going to be admitted to a single room. Hospital staff do recognize the needs of patients for privacy and all beds have curtains which pull round for bathing or if you have to use a bedpan. You will be encouraged to be up and about as quickly as possible so that you can make your own way to the bathroom.

Q **I always find hospital wards so depressing, mostly because everyone is sitting around in their nightclothes all day. Is this really necessary?**

A Many hospitals are now realizing that today's casual clothes, like tracksuits for example, are really no different from pyjamas and much more sensible to wear in the daytime. Check with the sister in charge of the ward before you are admitted to see if they will permit this.

Q **I have always been worried that if I have to go into hospital for an operation they will get me muddled up with someone else and I will have the wrong thing done. Is this possible?**

A It is certainly very, very unlikely because almost all hospitals use a wrist-band of some kind with your name and details on it. This enables anyone to check your identity, even when you are unconscious. As a further safeguard, you should check that the houseman or sister visits you before the operation and marks your body with an indelible pen — for example if your left leg is being operated on that limb should be marked at the point where the operation will take place. Make sure this is always done.

Q **I have now had two minor operations and have been violently sick after each one. It really is most unpleasant and I would like to know if there is anything that can be done about it?**

A Yes, you should talk to the anaesthetist and give details of your past history. It should be possible to give you an injection of an anti-nauseant drug at the same time as you are given the anaesthetic.

2
Healthy breasts

When the breasts begin to develop during puberty, they are a symbol both of sexuality and nurturing. The function of the breasts is to provide milk for a baby but they are also perceived to be a very vital part of a woman's attractiveness, both to herself and others. Any problems that affect the breasts can have a profound effect on a woman's view of herself, her confidence and self-esteem.

Nipples

Q **I have a large number of hairs around my nipples, which I find very embarrassing. Is this normal?**

A This is a constant source of misery to many women, but it is almost as common as having no such hair. Any of the usual hair removing techniques can be used on them, but plucking is not recommended as it sometimes stimulates more growth. Hair around the nipple has nothing to do with abnormal hormones or changing sex, but like facial and leg hair it is probably an inherited family or racial characteristic.

Q **I have had inverted nipples since I was a child, does this mean that I will not be able to breastfeed?**

A This is not an uncommon problem — many young girls' nipples are like this, and it is not until adult life that they need any attention. It will probably not affect your ability to breastfeed providing you take action to correct it during your pregnancy by wearing breast shields.

Q **What are breast shields and how do you use them?**

A These are made of rubber or plastic and worn under your bra, next to your skin. There is a small hole in the centre of them and the nipple is gently pulled through this by suction. You would start by wearing them for just a couple of hours a day at first and gradually increase the time towards the end of your pregancy. If this fails to bring out the nipples then you may not be able to feed.

Q **I have inverted nipples. How can I get them to turn out normally?**

A There are two things you can try. The first is the Hoffman technique which you could carry out two or three times a day. You first stretch the nipple by placing a finger on either side of your aerola and exerting gentle pressure on it. Then move your fingers so they are above and below the nipple and repeat as before. Breast shields are another method, and a full description is given in the previous question.

Q **I have had inverted nipples for many years and have tried most things without success. What else can be done to help?**

A It is possible to operate on inverted nipples that have not responded to any treatment. The tissue that tethers them in will be cut. But remember, unless you specifically want to breast feed, it really doesn't matter whether your nipples are inverted or not.

Q **One of my nipples has started to turn inwards. Should I worry about it?**

A You should consult your doctor at once. It is not normal for adult nipples to do this and it needs investigating.

Q **I have never been pregnant, but recently my nipples seem to be constantly weeping a sort of milk-like substance. Is this normal? I am 30 years old and on the Pill.**

A This is a condition called galactorrhoea, or inappropriate lactation. Although you are on the Pill you should make quite sure that this method of contraception has not failed you because galactorrhoea is usually caused by pregnancy.

Q **I know I'm not pregnant but my nipples are leaking milk. It is so embarrassing. What can be done about it?**

A Do visit your doctor who will check your blood for the presence of the hormone prolactin. If too much of it shows up, then this is what is causing the leaking. You will then need further tests to see why you are producing so much of this hormone. Some drugs can cause prolactin to be overproduced but the Pill is not one of them.

Q **Why do my nipples become hard in the cold, or when I'm sexually stimulated?**

A Most women's nipples are very sensitive to changes in temperature or to touch. The small muscle fibres within each nipple contract when they are stimulated and this has the effect of making the nipple erect.

Q **What does skin cancer look like? I have some brown, scab-like blemishes on and around my left nipple. I was wondering if this is anything serious? The right nipple is similarly affected, but does not look quite so bad.**

A It is extremely unusual to get skin cancer around a nipple. However, there is a condition called Paget's disease which affects the nipple. It looks like eczema and bleeds easily and if you think this is what you have, then it should be treated by a specialist. There could be a simpler explanation, though. The scab-like blemishes sound as though they are an encrustation caused by skin oils. If you use a softening skin lotion they should just lift off, but if you are worried then do consult your doctor.

Q **I started taking the Pill recently and my nipples have changed colour. Is this usual?**

A In fair-skinned women the nipples may become brown and pigmented as a side effect of your taking the Pill. This is quite normal. Exactly the same thing happens naturally to a lot of women when they first become pregnant.

Breasts

Q **Where can I get information on carrying out breast examination?**

A You can usually get an instruction leaflet from your local clinic or doctor, or a women's health care organization. The latter may also have a video that you can watch to make the procedure clearer.

Q **What do I look for when I carry out a breast self-examination?**

A There are several things you should check for, but basically you are looking for any change to the normal condition of your breasts. This can be in the size or shape of the breast itself, including any veins that are more prominent than usual or any skin that is a different texture. Or it may be a change in the nipple, possibly a discharge or bleeding. Remember it is a change from what is normal for *you*.

Q **My doctor has told me I've got mastitis. Could you explain exactly what this is?**

A Mastitis, or inflammation of the breasts, is a very common condition in women who have functioning ovaries. It usually occurs just before a period and is the response of the small breast glands to the hormones being produced by your ovaries. It is not usually due to any infection.

Q **Is there anything I can do for myself to help with mastitis?**

A As a first line measure, try wearing a comfortable but firm bra day and night during the times when you have this problem. This helps to prevent swelling of the breast. Eliminate caffeine from your diet during your premenstrual week, which means no coffee, tea or cola. Take vitamin B6 in a dose of up to 100mg a day for the second half of your cycle; although it is more commonly used to ease premenstrual tension it also helps many women with painful breasts.

Q **What help can my doctor give me for mastitis?**

A Talk to your doctor about the problem and there are several ways s/he may be able to help. Some women have their pain relieved by taking an oral contraceptive, but if this is not suitable for you then an anti-hormone preparation like Bromocryptine may be valuable, but only if your mastitis is so troublesome that it interferes with your daily routine.

Breast size and shape

Q **I have always been very flat-chested. Is there any exercise I can do to make my bust any bigger?**

A Not your actual bust, no. That is determined by your own hormones and the body build you inherited. Exercise can make your bust appear bigger, but it is the muscles which support the bust that you are developing. Good posture also helps your bust look bigger and exercise can assist there too.

Q **One of my breasts is larger than the other. Can I do anything about it?**

A This is extremely common; most women do not have breasts that are exactly the same size. The only way of evening them up would be with plastic surgery and it is unlikely you would want to go to such lengths for something that is not really a medical problem. A simple solution is to pad your bra to redress the balance.

Q **Older women often seem to have very droopy breasts. What causes this?**

A The breasts are given firmness and support by fibrous bands which attach and support the breast to the chest muscles. These ligaments lose some of their elasticity as we get older and so the breasts can lose their firmness.

Q **My breasts seem to change shape throughout the month. Is this normal?**

A Yes, it is common to most women throughout their monthly cycle, though it is more pronounced in some than others. The breasts usually feel more sensitive at ovulation (two weeks before the next period) and then again just before the period is due they may feel swollen and lumpy. It's due to the changing levels of the hormones oestrogen and progesterone, which return to normal levels once the period has started. This has the effect of returning the breasts to their usual size.

Q **I have very small breasts. Will I ever be able to breastfeed a baby?**

A The size and shape of the breast is not a critical factor. The bodily changes that occur during pregnancy allow most women to be able to breastfeed. In fact, women with small breasts are often much more successful at feeding than women with very large breasts.

Q **I have very large breasts which have been a constant source of embarrassment all my life. If I have them reduced will I still be able to breastfeed?**

A Reducing breast size is a complicated procedure and should not be undertaken without a great deal of thought and counselling. If you want to be able to breastfeed in the future then you must make that very clear to the surgeon so that extra care can be taken not to remove too much secretory tissue or cut through the major mammary ducts. Why not postpone the operation until you have completed your family, then both you and your surgeon will have an easier time.

Q **My doctor has agreed that I can have breast reduction surgery. What exactly is involved?**

A Ask your surgeon to draw you a diagram of exactly what s/he plans to do. There are several different surgical approaches and s/he will use the one best suited to your size and shape. The nipple is always left intact and attached to the breast tissue. It can then be mobilized and placed in a new opening on the breast skin to set it in the perfect place. Excess breast tissue is usually removed from the lower half of the breast. Do make sure you fully understand the operation. It usually gives excellent results, but as with all operations things can sometimes go wrong.

Q **How long would I have to stay in hospital after a breast reduction operation?**

A Surgeons vary in their advice, but in general, with no complications you could expect to be in hospital for up to three or four days. You would convalesce at home and then be ready, with care, to resume your normal routine in a week or two when the stitches had been removed and the scar had healed properly.

Screening

Q **I am 23 and have a worry about breast cancer. I have been to the hospital several times and they have told me that the small lumps in my breasts are only lumps of fat, but I should still check them regularly. I am not sure when to do this and how will I know when one is cancerous?**

A Any lump that comes and goes with the menstrual cycle is not related in any way to breast cancer. Your doctor or family planning clinic will show you how to carry out self-examination and this is usually best done in the week following menstruation.

Q **My company offers regular mammography screening but I have been too embarrassed to go. What exactly does it involve?**

A It is a very straightforward procedure. An X-ray is taken of your breasts and the female radiographer will explain to you exactly what you have to do, so there is no need to be embarrassed. You simply stand while your breast is evened out and smoothed by flattening it between two perspex plates. The X-ray is then taken. Because breasts vary in their sensitivity some women find this procedure a little uncomfortable, but for the vast majority there is no discomfort at all.

Q **I was recently screened for breast cancer and have been asked to go back. Does this mean they have found cancer?**

A Mammography X-rays show up tiny alterations in the breast which are impossible to detect on physical examination. The majority of these problems turn out not to be cancer but without further tests this is impossible to decide. Many women screened will need to be recalled for extra X-rays and more tests. Almost every one of these will turn out *not* to have breast cancer. However a very few, between four and eight women in every 1000, will have their cancers detected *early* by this means. Although it is no guarantee of complete cure, the earlier you can find a breast cancer then the better are your long-term prospects.

Cancer — surgery

Q **I have agreed to go into hospital for some exploratory surgery on my breast. I am anxious that the surgeon could remove my breast without my consent. How can I make sure this doesn't happen?**

A Once you are in hospital for your operation you will be asked to sign a consent form. It allows the surgeon to carry out an *agreed* operation, and agreed is the important word. The consent form must contain a written description of the operation that is planned, but sometimes this can be left rather open. In the case of breast abnormalities the operation may be described as 'breast biopsy and proceed as necessary'. The 'and proceed' to the surgeon may mean mastectomy and you must ask him or her to make clear exactly what s/he intends to do. If necessary you can adjust the words on the form and stipulate 'breast biopsy only' so both you and the surgeon are clear that s/he cannot proceed any further than that in this particular operation.

Q **I have cancer and the surgeon wants to remove one of my breasts. I am very proud of my figure and dread any disfigurement. Is there anything that can be done?**

A A large number of cancer surgeons will perform implant surgery on suitable patients and this can return your breast to almost its former appearance. You may even be offered this at the same time as the actual mastectomy operation. However you should bear in mind that with any implant there is always the risk of the body rejecting it.

Q **What exactly does a synthetic implant consist of?**

A It is a bag of liquid silicone which has very much the same consistency as breast tissue at body temperature. Once in place it is covered by your own skin and a new nipple can also be constructed, using a skin graft from other parts of the body.

Q **The surgeon has suggested that after my operation for cancer breast reconstruction could be carried out. What would that involve?**

A Breast reconstruction is carried out by using tissue from another part of your body to recreate a breast shape. Often, part of one of the big muscles from your back is used and tucked under the skin on the front of the chest wall to restore the shape of the breast. One advantage of this type of reconstruction is that it carries no risk of being rejected, as can happen with an implant.

Q **My 82 year old grandmother has just been found to have breast cancer. It is fairly small and she's very opposed to having any operation at all. Is this possible?**

A It is certainly quite possible and proper to treat some forms of breast cancer without an operation. X-ray treatment alone has been known to have very good results, and St George's Hospital in London has been treating women over 70 with a simple daily anti-hormone tablet which can be taken at home. Whatever your grandmother decides she should discuss the whole matter thoroughly with her doctor so that s/he can arrange for her referral to a suitable unit for consultation.

Q **It is possible that I may have to have a mastectomy and I am confused because my surgeon has talked about a 'partial' mastectomy. What would be left?**

A What your surgeon probably meant was a quadrantectomy. It means that s/he is going to remove the quarter of the breast that has the cancer in it, and leave the rest. This is usually possible when the cancer is on the outer, or arm-side, of the breast. S/he will probably take a few glands from the armpit at the same time. However, three quarters of your breast and the nipple can be left behind, because the pre-operative X-ray (mammogram) that you had showed that all this tissue was healthy.

Q **What is the difference between a simple and a radial mastectomy?**

A When a radial mastectomy is carried out the muscles of the chest wall are removed, along with the breast and lymph glands in the armpit. A simple mastectomy leaves these muscles intact.

Q **What is a subcutaneous mastectomy?**

A In a subcutaneous mastectomy the surgeon will take away almost all of the internal breast tissue but without disturbing the nipple and surrounding skin. It is usually carried out as a preventative procedure where there is a high risk of malignancy, but no actual cancer at present. To restore the shape of the breast an implant will be inserted at the same time.

Q **I know I have to have a mastectomy but I am concerned about the practical aspect. How do I buy bras and dresses, that kind of thing?**

A Talk first to your doctor to get all the information you need and then ask about local support groups. Your doctor may have information on one or your surgeon or hospital can often provide such help.

Q **After my mastectomy how should I take care of myself when I get home?**

A It is most important to try to get back to a normal way of life, and friends and family can be a great help here. On the physical side, you need to ensure that the shoulder on the affected side gets moving as quickly and as fully as possible so that you don't allow it to become stiff. However, you do need to protect the arm and hand on the affected side. Have blood tests taken from the 'good' arm and always wear gloves for gardening, washing up and any rough work. This is because surgery and radiotherapy frequently interfere with the lymphatic drainage of the arm on the same side as the breast cancer. In normal use this is not a problem, but if there is an infection of the arm through a cut or graze then it could cause a great deal of discomfort. There may well be a leaflet available which gives you all the information you need. Your local cancer group will be able to advise you.

Q **I had breast cancer ten years ago and had a mastectomy. I recovered completely but now have severe swelling in the arm on that side. What should I do?**

A First you must go and have your condition checked by your doctor. It is important to establish that there is no sign of any new cancer. Even though you have been disease free for ten years it is just possible that this new swelling is related not to the operation, but to a new problem. Once cancer has been excluded then you can look at managing this swelling, which is called lymphoedema.

Q **How can I treat lymphoedema?**

A Lymphoedema is tissue swelling and can occur anywhere. The swelling is due to retained fluid in the lymphatic system. After a mastectomy lymphoedema of the arm on the affected side is not uncommon. To reduce it, these suggestions should help. When you are sitting, keep your elbow on the arm rest, with your hand above it. When walking about, a simple sling may help reduce the swelling. Special inflatable cuffs can be used to encase the whole arm and massage the swelling away. These cuffs are used for a few minutes each hour or so. Your local cancer self-help group will have details.

Cancer — treatment

Q **I am to have radiation therapy for cancer of the breast. I am concerned about this because I thought radiation was dangerous.**

A Radiation can be both good and bad for you. It is bad in that gross exposure (as happened at Hiroshima and, more recently, Chernobyl) will kill all rapidly dividing cells in our bodies. This includes the blood cells and cells on the surface of the gut. If this happens we will die very quickly. At lower doses we will become very sick, but probably recover. But that same radiation, properly controlled and directed specifically against cancer cells, and given in infinitely lower doses, is a very effective way to stop the rapid growth of a large number of cancers that occur in human beings. Not all types of cancer are sensitive to radiation and there is also a limit to the amount of radiation treatment which can be given to any cancer sufferer. But breast cancer responds very well indeed to proper dosage.

Q **I have had surgery for breast cancer and am about to have a course of radiotherapy. Can you tell me what are the possible side-effects of this?**

A Side-effects from this type of treatment will not affect everyone in the same way, or to the same degree. Tiredness and depression are common reactions, both during the treatment and after it; the skin surrounding the area being treated may become red and sore which can last for some weeks afterwards. Women with light complexions (especially those with red hair) are more sensitive to this effect. Another effect on the skin is that it can change colour. Although the skin usually returns to its normal shade after treatment it can remain permanently lighter, or darker, than the surrounding skin area. Underarm hair will fall out as a result of treatment, but it will grow back eventually.

Q **When I have radiotherapy I am worried about my skin becoming sore. What can I do to prevent this?**

A With modern radiotherapy machines and the newer types of treatment it is very rare to get any serious skin soreness. Your radiotherapist will be able to advise you and give more individual information. As a self-help measure, if your skin is uncomfortable then aloe vera juice applied straight onto the skin can help alleviate the discomfort and help it to heal.

Q **I had breast surgery last year, followed by radiotherapy. Now my consultant has suggested chemotherapy, but what exactly does this involve?**

A It is treatment by drugs that usually will involve a programme over six months or a year. It is a long process because time must be allowed for the body to recover between each treatment. A variety of drugs will be given, each having its own particular effect.

Q **Do I have to go into hospital for chemotherapy?**

A It is usual for the treatment to take place in hospital so that the drugs, and any possible side-effects, can be thoroughly monitored. However if you have the facilities, and the doctor is willing, then you could be treated at home, especially if your chemotherapy is by tablets rather than by injection.

Q **How are the drugs administered in chemotherapy treatment?**

A It will depend on your individual treatment, but there are a number of possibilities. They can be given orally in tablet form, by injection, or straight into a vein either by injection or by using a drip.

Q **What are the side-effects of chemotherapy?**

A They will depend very much on the particular drugs used and the dosage that you are given. Susceptibility will vary from one individual to another, but these drugs do affect all cells in the body and therefore can have a wide range of side-effects. Amongst those commonly reported are mouth ulcers, nausea and vomiting, constipation and diarrhoea, hair loss, lowered blood count, cessation of periods, menopausal symptoms, weight gain and depression.

Q **The side-effects for chemotherapy are rather frightening, there seem so many of them. Will I get all of them?**

A With any treatment it is important to remember that each person reacts differently. You may get none, or just a few side-effects, but certainly not all of them at any one time. Your doctor will adjust the dosage so that you have the fewest possible side-effects consistent with a proper dose of the drugs.

Q **I have just had an operation for breast cancer and I've been told I am to take hormones for the rest of my life. I thought hormones were bad for breasts?**

A You have probably been prescribed Tamoxifen, an anti-oestrogen preparation which is valuable, particularly for women with breast cancer which appears after the menopause. Very few, if any, side-effects are reported in the vast majority of women.

3
Healthy menstruation and sex

The years from puberty until the menopause are among the most important in a woman's life. It is the time of the greatest bodily changes and when some of the biggest challenges to good health can occur.

Menstruation

Q **I am 15 years old and my periods have not started yet. All my friends already have theirs, so what is wrong with me?**

A Nothing at all, you are just developing at a different rate from your friends and that is perfectly normal. Periods can start at any age between nine and 16 years, so there is no need for you to be concerned for at least another year. However you should by now have experienced some changes, such as developing a bust and the growth of some hair on your body. Do try and discuss your anxiety with your mother or an older woman friend.

Q **The doctor says my daughter has an imperforate hymen. What does this mean?**

A The hymen, or maidenhead, is a thin film of tissue which separates the vagina from the outside world. Usually there is a gap in it so that menstrual blood can escape, and this gap is made wider at the time of first sexual intercourse. An imperforate hymen has no opening at all, and therefore no way for menstrual blood to escape from the body. In cases like that of your daughter it is necessary to open the hymen by a small operation. When the hymen heals it then has a gap in it which will allow her to have normal periods in future.

Q **I have a 17 year old daughter who has been menstruating regularly for two years. Her periods have gradually stopped over the last few months and she is also losing a lot of weight. She seems quite lively and doesn't want to go to the doctor, but should I insist?**

A The clue here may be her loss of weight. It is possible that she may be anorexic, because one of the first things to go in this condition are the periods. Try to persuade, rather than insist, that she sees a doctor because her condition should be checked out. Do watch carefully what she *actually* eats — not what she says she eats.

Q **About a week before my period is due I get a dark line across the top of my lip. It looks like a moustache and only fades slightly when my period is over. What is causing it?**

A There is a condition called chloasma, which is an increased pigmentation of the skin of the face and other parts of the body. It is often associated with pregnancy, but also with women taking the oral contraceptive pill. The places it appears are on the upper lip, across the forehead, round the nipples and in a straight line stretching down from the navel. The only way to treat it is to stop taking the Pill or disguise the line with make up.

Q **It feels like I lose a lot of blood during a period. How much is the average?**

A Generally around one fluid ounce, or two tablespoonfuls. If you lose more than this, say over three ounces, or 80ml, then this would be termed menorrhagia, or excessive loss. However the blood is diluted with a lot of mucus material, so that it may seem that you lose a lot more than this.

Q **What are the causes of period pain?**

A Pain related to menstruation is called dysmenorrhea and there are two main types. 'Primary' affects young girls within a year or two of starting their periods, usually when ovulation begins to take place. 'Secondary' dysmenorrhea can start at any time of life but usually occurs after several years of normal pain-free periods. The cause may be due to a variety of conditions including fibroids, ovarian cysts or endometriosis.

Q **Are painful periods a normal part of a woman's life?**

A On the first day or two of a period many women experience some discomfort, but any pain which keeps you away from your normal occupation should be reported to your doctor for proper investigation and treatment.

Q **What treatment is there for painful periods?**

A First you must see your doctor to exclude any physical cause for the pain. Once this is done, then the most simple and effective way of stopping period pain is to suppress the ovaries and prevent an egg from maturing. This can be done by taking the Pill. An alternative is to take progestogen in the second half of the monthly cycle, but your doctor will be able to advise which is best for you. If you prefer, and the pain is not too great, then you could try a painkiller such as ibuprofen or paracetamol and that may be sufficient.

Q **I am a very keen runner and am out training most days. Although I am very fit and healthy my periods have stopped completely, and I am sure I am not pregnant. What has caused it?**

A If you are certain you are not pregnant — and it is still the most common reason for a missed period — then the most likely explanation is that you are taking too much exercise. Although it is an excellent thing to be fit, excessive exercise can give rise to problems. It causes a substantial drop in hormone levels and this is enough to cause your periods to stop. Also, as well as disturbing the menstrual cycle, excessive exercise can lead to thinning of the bones — osteoporosis.

Irregular bleeding

Q Although my periods have been fairly normal for the last few years, just recently I have been suffering very heavy bleeding. I am now 48, so is this a sign of the menopause?

A Continuous, heavy or painful bleeding is *not* a sign of the menopause and must be reported to your doctor and investigated. It is almost always due to quite innocent conditions, but this type of bleeding can lead to quite severe anaemia.

Q Endometriosis is something I have suffered from for the last two years, but my doctor doesn't seem to be able to help. What exactly is it?

A Endometriosis occurs when some cells of the womb lining settle in other parts of the abdomen. Then each month, responding to the normal hormonal changes, these cells break down and there is a small amount of bleeding from the associated blood vessels — just like in menstruation. However in this case there is nowhere for the blood to go, so it collects just like a bruise. As the blood liquefies it may give rise to a sticky, painful cyst which gets stuck onto other things, like the gut. Blood is also intensely irritating to the peritoneum, so many sufferers experience a mini peritonitis each month.

Q Is there a typical 'type' who is likely to suffer from endometriosis?

A It is confined to women in their reproductive years and is most common in those in their thirties. Childlessness, for whatever reason, also seems to make women more likely to be sufferers.

Q I think I have endometriosis because I have similar symptoms to my sister who had it ten years ago. She was told to just go away and have a baby, but surely there is other treatment available now?

A Having a baby was the advice that was given, because a full nine months without any periods did often cause the endometriosis to burn itself out. Even if you have the same symptoms as your sister you cannot assume that you have endometriosis without going to the doctor for proper investigation. If you do have this condition, then there is now a nine month course of hormone treatment available, as well as drugs which suppress the pituitary gland. These can be used in the more difficult cases. Not every woman wants, or can have, a baby just to treat endometriosis.

Pre-menstrual syndrome

Q In articles I have read both PMS and PMT are regularly referred to. Which is correct?

A They are just different names for the same thing, so you can use whichever you prefer. PMS stands for pre-menstrual *syndrome*, and PMT means pre-menstrual *tension*. Generally, PMS is the term most used by doctors as it gathers together a whole group of symptoms, not all of which are related specifically to tension.

Q **Does every woman get pre-menstrual symptoms?**

A Most women do get some warning signs from their body when the next period is about to happen: some get breast tenderness, sleeplessness, constipation or swelling of the abdomen. Unfortunately, for possibly as many as 10 per cent, the week or two before a period can give rise to very real problems in the shape of PMS.

Q **Why do I suffer badly from PMS while my younger sister doesn't?**

A Though PMS can strike any woman of menstruating age, it is usually more common to suffer from it first in the mid-thirties. No one knows the exact cause of PMS and so it is impossible to say why one person suffers and another doesn't. It is believed that it is something to do with an imperfect balance of hormones or vitamins in the body, but a complete solution is still a long way off.

Q **Since I began my new job my PMS has got worse. I now do a lot of travelling and don't always have time for proper meals. Could this have made any difference?**

A Yes, it could. Stress certainly doesn't help and irregular meals may be making it worse. PMS is often aggravated by low blood sugar levels, so it is important to eat regularly — preferably with no more than three hours between meals. If this is really impossible for you then you may get relief by carrying snacks that are high in protein or complex carbohydrate, so that your blood sugar level remains stable. This will help with those symptoms such as headaches, nervousness, irritability and food cravings. But do make sure you don't overeat — otherwise this will give you problems for the other three weeks of your cycle!

Q **Every month I suffer from very bad PMS. I seem to shake a lot and I also get very thirsty. I talked to my doctor and he suggested that I cut down on the amount of tea I have. I drink up to 20 cups a day, but how will cutting down on that help my PMS?**

A Anyone who is as thirsty as you are certainly does need to talk to their doctor about it because it can be a symptom of a type of diabetes. In your case, the amount of caffeine you are taking in could well be precipitating your PMS and certainly will be making it worse. Caffeine is a potent stimulant, present in tea as well as in coffee, and five or six cups of either is probably the maximum amount anyone should have in a day. Caffeine is also present in cola drinks.

Q **What can I do to help myself with my PMS symptoms?**

A Taking additional vitamin B6 and Evening Primrose Oil has helped many women with PMS and it is also worth looking at what you eat. Sugar, chocolate, caffeine and alcohol have proved to be triggers for PMS in some cases and it may be worth eliminating them from your diet and seeing whether it makes any difference to your symptoms.

Q **What treatment can my doctor offer me for PMS?**

A There is no universal 'cure' because there are no universal symptoms. For some it is an actual physical condition, for others it is more an emotional state. Some women find that taking the Pill removes all problems because it stops ovulation. For others, taking the hormone progesterone in the second half of the menstrual cycle may be the most effective treatment.

Sex

Q I bled quite heavily when I first had sexual intercourse. What caused it and what should I have done about it?

A A small blood loss on first intercourse is quite common and is associated with a torn hymen. This is the flap of skin across the entrance to the vagina and the blood comes from little blood vessels, or capillaries, which are in the actual tissue of the hymen. The best way to treat such bleeding is to apply firm pressure, either by sitting on your fist or an ice pack, even though the area may be tender. If the bleeding continues it may be necessary to go to the casualty department of your local hospital.

Q I have not had a sexual partner since my husband died 15 years ago. I am about to be married again, but am worried that I will find sex difficult and painful.

A For the older woman, and those who have not had intercourse for some years, the introitus can shrink and become smaller. Lubrication of the vagina may be lacking and this could cause some problems during intercourse. Additional lubrication can be given with the use of KY Jelly, and you can buy this over the counter at a pharmacy. Using an oestrogen vaginal cream, under your doctor's instructions, can help the tissues relax and become more supple.

Q **I have been using a hormone cream for the last couple of years for dryness of the vagina. Does continued use of it have any serious side-effects such as cervical cancer?**

A As far as is known at present, there is no cancer risk from using a vaginal hormone cream. However, you should continue to have cervical smears every three to five years — or more frequently if your doctor advises it — until you are aged 65 and have had a series of clear smears.

Q **When I make love I find that I am rather dry and this is uncomfortable. A friend has said that baby oil is a good lubricant and I was wondering whether to try it.**

A Baby oils and some petroleum jelly preparations can be a bit messy on the bedclothes. Also, if you use a sheath or diaphragm for contraception, these substances can weaken the latex rubber. Use KY Jelly instead, it has a water-soluble base and does not seem to have the same damaging effect on the cap or sheath.

Q **Every time I make love, I get a slight bleeding. Is this anything to worry about?**

A If you get bleeding after sex, other than the very first time, then you should definitely get it checked by your doctor. It may be nothing to worry about at all, but it would be better to be certain.

Q   **I am in my early fifties and had a womb scrape last year after I had some bleeding after sex. I was told to go back to my GP if it happened again and he gave me some cream to use. It hasn't recurred, but I am worried I may have a cancer that is not being treated.**

A   If no serious abnormality was found when you had the womb scrape then you don't have cancer now. What probably happened is that the lining of the vagina was lacking in the hormone oestrogen. This naturally happens after the menopause and in some women gives rise to a vagina which is easily bruised by sexual intercourse. If the bleeding does recur then go back and see your doctor again. If not then forget it.

Tests

Q   **My doctor wants me to have a smear test. Does this mean he thinks I have cancer?**

A   The smear test is not a test for cancer; it is a test for *pre-cancer*. Your doctor is not singling you out, this is a simple procedure that should be regularly carried out on every woman up to the age of 65. Cervical cancer is almost entirely preventable, but only if every woman agrees to have a regular smear test.

Q   **I have just had my first-ever smear test at the age of 48. My doctor has written to ask me to visit the surgery as the test is abnormal. I am worried sick about this, what does it mean?**

A   It means that you will probably need some further investigations, but it doesn't mean that you have cancer. The chances are that you have a pre-cancerous condition of the neck of the womb and this can be treated quite simply in the gynaecological out-patient department.

Q **How often should I have a smear test?**

A Every sexually active woman needs regular tests at least every three to five years, starting at the age of 25, if not before. Tests can be arranged by contacting your doctor, health visitor or Family Planning Clinic.

Q **I had a smear test recently and have just been recalled for another one. Why have they done this?**

A Abnormal smears are more common among women in the 25 to 34 age group, and of every 100 that show up abnormal the likelihood is that less than 15 of these women would eventually develop a real cervical cancer — even if they had no treatment. The trouble is it is not possible to identify exactly *which* 15 women out of the 100 are at real risk so treatment must be offered to all women with an abnormal smear. Occasionally, the smear test can be altered by a mild vaginal infection and women are then recalled for early repeat smears. This is merely a precaution and nothing at all to get worried about.

Q **I have just had an abnormal smear test. The doctor has said that it isn't cancer but they still want to treat me and do follow-up tests. Is this really necessary?**

A Just because it is not cancer at this stage does not mean that it can be ignored. It is a warning and it is vital to have any treatment suggested. If left untreated it could develop into cancer after several years and this is too big a risk to take. Treatment and follow-up tests are entirely in your own best interests.

Q **My doctor thinks I might have fibroids and wants to send me for an ultrasound. What is this exactly?**

A It is a way of looking within your body by using sound waves. These waves are processed through a computer and appear on a video screen. Photographs can be taken of this picture to create a permanent record. It is a commonly used diagnostic tool and many people are fascinated to see the 'map' of their body which appears on the screen.

Q **Is ultrasound painful?**

A No, not at all. There is no pain or discomfort involved. What happens is that you lie down comfortably and a technician will put some lubricating substance over the area that is to be looked at. This ensures that the sound waves connect properly with your skin and are not dispersed through an air gap. A sound 'pad' is gently smoothed back and forth across your skin. It sends sound waves into your body and picks up the echoes.

Surgical procedures

Q **What is a biopsy?**

A It is a procedure for identifying a disease or abnormality by taking a small fragment of tissue which can be looked at under the microscope later. A biopsy is usually a minor surgical procedure and can be done without anaesthetic in some situations, for example biopsying the cervix. For other tissue samples, like the ovary, a general anaesthetic is necessary. Once the biopsy has been studied by the specialist then it is possible to make decisions about what treatment will be necessary.

Q **I have been having a lot of abdominal pain recently and I have been told I am going to have a laparoscopy. Just what is this?**

A It is a procedure to enable the surgeon to have a look into your abdomen to see just what may be causing your problem. A small incision is made just below the navel and a long narrow 'torch' is inserted. Gas is used to lift up the abdominal wall so that the womb, uterus and Fallopian tubes are seen clearly. Instruments can be passed down through the laparoscope to take biopsies of different tissues, to to carry out sterilization. The incision is so small it can be closed with one stitch.

Q **I am to have a hysterectomy quite soon and I would like to find out as much as possible about it, before I have the operation.**

A It is always a good idea to have as much information as possible before any surgical procedure. Your surgeon or doctor will answer any questions you may have and you could ask them to put you in touch with other patients who have had this operation.

Q **What is the difference between a hysterectomy and a total hysterectomy?**

A There is no difference. These operations are the same. However, in a sub-total hysterectomy the cervix (neck of the womb) is left behind.

Q Is a hysterectomy really necessary?

A hysterectomy is a major operation and is not recommended lightly. If the operation is being carried out because of pain or bleeding associated with periods, or for prolapse or urinary problems, then you are the one who is the best judge of whether it is necessary. You must weigh whether the present discomfort and pain is sufficient for you to seek the relief that the operation will bring. If the hysterectomy is being recommended for treating cancer of the cervix or womb, then you really do not have a choice. The operation is necessary and total recovery from this type of cancer is very common if treated at an early stage.

Q Is it always essential to remove the ovaries when a hysterectomy is carried out?

No, in fact the ovaries are usually left behind. However, if you are past the menopause then surgeons often prefer to remove the ovaries as well because they can be another potential source of trouble. If you have not yet reached the menopause then, always assuming that they are normal, one or both of the ovaries may be left to produce its natural hormones. This may not be possible if cancer is present. Your surgeon should always fully discuss *all* the options with you before your operation.

Q What kind of scar will I have after a hysterectomy?

It depends on how the operation is carried out. The womb can be removed from above, through an incision in the abdomen, or from below, through the vagina. The decision is up to the surgeon, but you may be able to state whether you prefer a bikini scar running across your abdomen or a vertical scar from the navel downwards.

Q I had a hysterectomy about a month ago, and I would like to get my figure back into shape once I have fully recovered from the operation.

A The very best time to start to exercise is *before* the operation, but failing that it is a very good idea to start exercising as soon as you feel able to. There are many types of hysterectomy so there is no hard and fast rule about the amount of exercise you can properly undertake. Be guided initially by your surgeon and the physiotherapist or read one of the many excellent books written on this subject.

Q How soon can I resume normal lovemaking after a hysterectomy? I am feeling quite well again.

A It is always reassuring to a woman that her partner finds her attractive and it is very important after a hysterectomy that she is made to feel confident in her femininity. From this point of view the resumption of your sex life is vital. Some four to six weeks after the operation many women are comfortable enough to want to have normal, gentle intercourse but it is important that both partners are happy and comfortable and not afraid. Fear is a great turn off for the sex drive and such apprehension could spoil lovemaking for a long time if it is started before both of you have gained confidence.

Q I had a hysterectomy five years ago, leaving me with both ovaries, so why do I still have to have pelvic examinations?

A Although you have had a hysterectomy it is still important to check that your ovaries are not developing cysts or other problems which may need treatment.

Q **For what reasons are D & C operations carried out?**

A Dilation and Curettage — or D & C's — allow the surgeon to assess the size and shape of the womb and gather pieces of the lining for study under a microscope. Doctors don't always know exactly what is causing your symptoms and so a D & C is a way of making a thorough examination. It is often suggested for the treatment of painful or heavy periods, infertility, the non-appearance of periods in a young girl, and as a check on all irregular bleeding. It may be suggested for post-menopausal patients who experience bleeding, as it is the simplest and most thorough way of checking that there is no cancer present.

Q **I am due to go into hospital for a D & C and am worried if I have to be shaved for it. If so, I would rather do it at home in private. Is that allowed?**

A Most hospitals have abandoned shaving for simple procedures like D & C, and even for normal childbirth. It has been shown that shaving has no effect on whether you get an infection after the operation or not. In fact many people get skin rashes in the shaven area, which are much worse than any infection.

Q **I have a prolapsed womb and the surgeon is going to do a Manchester repair. What on earth is it?**

A Nothing very mysterious — it is simply a technique that got its name from being first developed in hospitals in Manchester. If you have a dropped womb, a tuck is taken in both the front and the back walls of the vagina, the ligaments supporting the neck of the womb are tightened and the neck of the womb (the cervix) is shortened.

Q It has been suggested that I have a vaginal repair operation. What is involved and is it really necessary?

A The vagina is supported by muscles which sling it from the pelvic bones in front, behind and around the sides. If there is any weakening of these muscles, and both pregnancy and the menopause are major factors, then the womb may be pushed down into the vagina or the bladder and rectum may also sag downwards. This is called a prolapse. The operation involves stitching the walls of the vagina back so that they regain their normal shape. Only you can decide, together with your surgeon, if the discomfort of your condition warrants an operation.

Q I am going into hospital for a prolapse operation. How soon will I be up and about again?

A Almost certainly you will be up and about the day after your operation and encouraged to go to the bathroom. You will probably be allowed to shower from day one, and have a bath after a day or so. After the operation it may be difficult to pass urine for the first few days and the nurses looking after you will take special care of this. All the stitches used in the vagina dissolve by themselves but there may be a few stitches on the outside if you are having a posterior repair. These will be removed seven to ten days after the operation. Most women are sent home or to a convalescent home after their hospital stay and, depending on the type of work you do, you may return to it about six to eight weeks after the operation.

Infections and diseases

Q I have an embarrassing itch around the outside of my vagina. I have had it for a while, though I don't have any discharge.

A There are many reasons why you could have such a problem. If you have recently taken a course of antibiotics you may have a fungus infection called thrush which can itch terribly. There is also a condition called pruritus vulvae which can occur after the menopause and seems to be caused by diminishing hormone levels. You should visit your doctor and, if necessary, you will be referred to a dermatologist who can advise you on further treatment.

Q What is the difference between candida and thrush?

A Candida, monilia and thrush are all names for the same condition and these names are interchangeable.

Q What causes thrush?

A It is caused by infection with a type of yeast, and the single most common cause of yeast infection is taking antibiotics. This is because the antibiotics kill not only the bacteria that are making us ill, but all the good bacteria which keep us healthy as well. If you are taking the Pill, are pregnant or a diabetic then you are also more vulnerable to yeast infections.

Q Can I do anything to prevent thrush?

A You can restrict those things that allow yeast to flourish, like antibiotics. Only take them when it is absolutely necessary. Sugar also plays a part in promoting the ideal conditions for thrush so try to cut it out of your diet. Yeasts also love moist, warm airless crevices so avoid tightly fitting pants, tights or trousers and avoid synthetic fabrics next to your skin.

Q Should I abstain from sex while I have thrush?

A Thrush infections can be passed from person to person and, where there is a vaginal yeast infection, it is important that your partner either uses a sheath until the treatment is completed, or is also treated.

Q What is the usual treatment for thrush?

A Vaginal thrush is treated by anti-fungal pessaries or creams used directly in the vagina.

Q After having treatment for thrush, what can I do to help myself?

A You need to replace the healthy intestinal flora that has been lost during treatment with antibiotics. Try to avoid the following: sugar, refined foods, 'blue' cheeses, wines, vinegar, bread, yeast, tea, and coffee. Increase your intake of fresh fruit and vegetables, and 'live' natural yoghurt, and try taking a supplement of yeast-free B complex and a course of acidophilus tablets.

Q **I enjoy having oral sex with my partner, but recently he has developed a cold sore round his mouth and I think he could pass this infection on to me. He says I am being silly, but am I right?**

A Cold sores are highly infectious. The virus particles present in the blisters, and the wet sores, can penetrate delicate tissue. Your partner could easily transmit the virus from his mouth to your vagina and thus infect you.

Q **What are the symptoms of genital herpes?**

A Around 50 per cent of people having their first infection will not have any symptoms at all. In its minor form, it comes out (just as it does around the mouth) as tender, sometimes itchy areas which within a day or two develop a crop of small water-filled blisters. These blisters break, a scab crusts over and dries out. The blisters are full of virus particles ready to be passed on to others and the scabs that form after the blisters can also contain large quantities of virus.

Q **I had genital herpes a few months ago and the doctor warned me that I may keep getting further attacks. What are the chances that I'll avoid it?**

A At least one in five patients never has another bout, and that figure may be as high as one in every two people. They are the lucky ones because for other sufferers herpes is a recurrent condition which may be brought on by an unrelated illness, general stress and tiredness or by nothing in particular that you can identify.

Q **How can I avoid getting genital herpes?**

A Never have intercourse when your partner has active herpes — this may sound obvious, but it is not always easy to tell as around 50 per cent of people have no symptoms with their first attack. The sheath, or condom, is a very good protective but the diaphragm is not.

Q **I think I have a wart on the skin outside my vagina. What can I do about it?**

A Warts are commonly found around the anus and lips of the vagina. They are contagious and can be contracted during sexual intercourse. The usual treatment is Podophyllin paint, in concentrations of 10 to 25 per cent. The wart is coated with this once a week and has to be washed off three or four hours later. If you have warts you should have regular cervical smears as the wart virus may be involved in the alteration of the cervical cells. Do check with your doctor or go to a special clinic to find out exactly what the problem is.

Q **Does the contraceptive sheath really give adequate protection against getting AIDS?**

A The sheath is one of the best methods of protection from the chance sexual contact. When it is used together with the spermicide nonoxynol, which also appears to work well against the AIDS virus, then this combination is very effective. You can get such combined product from many Family Planning Clinics or buy it over the counter at the chemist. However, the best protection against getting AIDS is to have sex with as few partners as possible.

Q I have had a severe vaginal itch for a week or so and when I went for an examination they said I had TV, but I didn't know what that meant.

A It stands for Trichomonas Vaginalis, which is a small one-celled creature which lives in the gut and is specially constructed so it can live without oxygen. The vagina is an ideal home for it to thrive and it is spread through sexual contact, so both you are your partner must have treatment so that reinfection does not occur.

Womb, ovaries and cervix

Q I seem to have a discharge from my vagina. I often get to work in the morning and find that my pants are damp, and I have to take a spare pair with me. What is causing this?

A It is possible that it is simply an excess of mucus which is normally produced around ovulation; wearing a panty liner would save you having to change your underwear so frequently. One other explanation might apply. If you have a bath every morning, and have good muscles, it is possible that some of the bath water is trapped in the vagina and it will then just leak out during the day.

Q I went to my doctor and, after having an number of tests, he has diagnosed polycystic ovary disease. What has caused this to happen?

A Polycystic ovary disease (PCOD) probably starts at adolescence. The hormone balance gets out of phase and the glandular part of the ovary is over-stimulated by hormones originating in the adrenal gland. This leads to an excess production of the substance which makes androgens, the male hormone. All women make male hormone, but in PCOD there is rather too much.

Q What treatment for PCOD is available?

A Blood tests can show special changes in the hormone pattern and ultrasound scanning provides very detailed information about the presence of cysts in the ovary. Once a diagnosis has been made, hormone treatment is usually prescribed — though just occasionally an operation is necessary to remove parts of the cystic ovary.

Q I have been told I have cervical erosion — does this mean I am wearing away?!

A No, it is one of those terms that has been in use by gynaecologists for a very long time but is actually nothing like it sounds. The word 'erosion' in this context simply means that the delicate lining of the cervical canal is found on the vaginal surface of the cervix. The surface of the canal looks much redder because it has a more prolific blood supply than the vaginal surface, and it was this appearance that originally suggested the term 'erosion'.

Q My 15 year old daughter has cervical erosion. I thought this only occurred in sexually active women, so does it mean she is having sexual intercourse?

A An erosion, more properly called a cervical ectopy, is the normal state just after puberty. At this time, the cervix changes shape and the delicate lining of the cervical canal 'pouts' onto the vaginal surface of the cervix. Erosion has nothing to do with sexual activity and can certainly occur in virgins.

Q **How can cervical erosion occur?**

A During childbirth the cervix often suffers small tears because it has to stretch to let the baby through. Later, the healing may be incomplete and the cervical canal may be exposed to the vagina to a greater or lesser degree. This is one cause of erosion, but others are given in the previous two questions.

Q **What are the symptoms of cervical erosion, and does it always have to be treated?**

A Treatment of a cervical erosion is only necessary if it is producing symptoms. These are increased vaginal discharge, irregular bleeding or infertility. Many women have cervical erosion and know nothing about it unless told so by their doctor. There is no need to have treatment unless it is causing any problems.

Q **How is cervical erosion treated?**

A The delicate tissue of the cervical canal is cauterized. The vaginal lining is then allowed to grow over and cover the scarred area. Cauterization can be by burning, freezing or using a laser on the affected area. All these techniques are equally effective and some have the advantage that they can be done in the out-patients' department, so saving you the upheaval of being admitted to hospital.

Q I had a hysterectomy two years ago but was left with my ovaries. Twice recently I have passed a large blood clot in my urine but my doctor was unable to find anything wrong when he carried out a urine test. What is causing this?

A After a hysterectomy there may be an area of proud flesh in the scar at the top of your vagina which bleeds occasionally and may need cauterizing. You will need to have a full internal examination to establish whether this is the cause and you should discuss this with your doctor.

Q I recently saw a gynaecologist who told me I had a polyp on my cervix. What does this mean?

A Polyps can occur anywhere in the body. They grow on sites where there are mucus-making glands. Some of these tiny glands overgrow to make an extra bit of flesh which then produces a lot more mucus than is absolutely necessary. On the cervix a polyp usually makes its presence known either by vaginal discharge or by irregular bleeding. Treatment is usually as an out-patient, but your gynaecologist may wish to take you in for a complete check by uterine curettage.

Q I was in hospital recently for a laparoscopy and the surgeon said I had adhesions. I didn't want to seem foolish by not knowing what he meant, so could you tell me?

A Adhesions are fibrous bands of tissue which are sometimes attached to other pieces of the gut, or to the side wall of the abdomen. After any operation on your abdomen, or any pelvic infection, sometimes scar tissue forms between two adjacent loops of bowel and tethers them to each other. Usually the body can cope without this causing problems, but sometimes it interferes with the normal mobility of the intestine and this will give rise to a colicky kind of pain.

Q When I had a pelvic examination recently, the doctor said I had fibroids. What are they?

A In between the muscle fibres of the womb are strands of fibrous tissue. If this tissue grows too much it creates round balls within the womb muscle and these are called fibroids. They vary enormously in size and can be as small as a little fingernail or as large as a baby. They are usually entirely innocent.

Q Who is most likely to get fibroids?

A They are slightly more common in women who have not had any children by their mid-thirties, and in black women compared with white women of the same age. They are also increasingly common as women get older. As many as 50 per cent of all women will have a fibroid or two by the time they are 50.

Q **Is it always necessary to have fibroids treated?**

A No, it depends on their size and where they are situated in the womb. Whether you need treatment will depend entirely on whether you have any symptoms that are causing you distress. It is essential however to have a proper diagnosis to rule out other conditions such as ovarian cysts which are pretending to be fibroids. Ovarian cysts almost always need treatment.

Q **My periods have got heavier and heavier recently and I have been told this is due to fibroids. Why do they cause this bleeding?**

A Your fibroids are probably growing under the inside lining of the womb which sheds each month in menstruation. They cause the bleeding surface to increase enormously and periods consequently become heavier. You probably have clots of blood each month as well. Fibroids in other situations in the womb may not cause any increased bleeding.

Q **Is it possible for fibroids to be cancerous?**

A The chances of a fibroid becoming malignant are very remote, but possible.

The menopause

Q **People talk a lot about the menopause but what exactly is it?**

A The menopause is the permanent stopping of the normal monthly blood flow. The periods may suddenly stop, or they may become progressively less and happen at increasingly long intervals. Several periods may be missed then they will restart and continue regularly for a few months, then stop again, hiccuping onwards to a final stop.

Q **At what age can I expect the menopause to start?**

A It can happen naturally at any time, but the average age in the UK is about 49 years old. Average means that half of all women will stop before this age and the other half will go on longer. It may also be related to the age at which your periods started. For some reason it seems that the younger you are when you start, the longer you go on menstruating past the average age.

Q **How can I tell if my irregular bleeding is a sign of the menopause or something else?**

A If you have any irregular vaginal bleeding which happens without rhyme or reason, it must *never* be considered due to the menopause. If you have heavy bleeding with clots, even if it does happen regularly; pain with periods, especially if this is a new thing; any bleeding that happens after sex, then these *may* be related to the menopause but can equally be due to lots of other things and *must* be checked by your doctor.

Q **What are the common symptoms of the menopause and does everyone get them?**

A The usual ones are flushing, particularly of the face, head and neck during the daytime; night sweats; and a dry vagina. It is possible to have none, or all of these symptoms. They may come one at a time or all together. Most women experience some symptoms but there are quite a few who have none at all.

What treatment is there for menopause sufferers?

 Menopause symptoms are usually due to a lack of hormones — the most common being low oestrogen levels. For this reason HRT (Hormone Replacement Therapy) is often prescribed but it is essential to have a thorough check-up before undertaking a course of treatment. Treatment will vary (depending on whether you have had a hysterectomy or not) but will usually involve giving the hormones oestrogen and progestogen in low doses.

 What form does HRT take?

It can be given in four ways; orally as tablets; by implantation under the skin; as patches of hormones stuck onto the skin; and, especially in Continental Europe, by injection. Oestrogen can also be given locally as a treatment to the vagina.

What menopausal symptoms can HRT help with?

It can help with the most common ones of hot flushes, night sweats and a dry vagina. On its own, HRT will not relieve other symptoms of the menopause such as depression, tiredness or lack of concentration. But by enabling you to get a good night's sleep, and by eliminating hot flushes, you may feel much more able to cope.

Q **Are there any procedures I have to go through before I can be prescribed HRT?**

A HRT may be prescribed and monitored by a specialist, or your personal doctor. They will want you to undergo a check-up which will include weight measurement, blood pressure and a cervical smear. They may also ask for thyroid function tests, blood tests for anaemia and serum cholesterol levels, and — of course — a mammagram which is part of your regular breast screening.

Q **If it is so helpful why isn't every woman prescribed HRT?**

A HRT is not a cure for menopausal symptoms, only a way of relieving some of them. Not every woman gets these problems.

Q **Is there any reason why my doctor wouldn't prescribe HRT for me?**

A There are some women whose medical history makes them unsuitable for HRT. Particularly those with severe heart disease, raised blood pressure, or a history of deep vein thrombosis. Women who have (or have had) cancer of the breast, cervix, uterus or ovaries will rarely be prescribed HRT.

Q **I was given a prescription for HRT last year and although my symptoms were helped a lot at the time, now they are back to where they were. Should I go and see my doctor again?**

A HRT only works as long as you take it. It does not make the menopausal symptoms go away, just alleviates the worst of them. You need to take it continuously to relieve symptoms. You should go back to your doctor for further consultation and prescription if you are still troubled.

Q **Although I am 55 my periods are still occurring fairly regularly. Is this usual?**

A Only a few women go on having periods so late in life and for those that do it is often recommended that they should have their womb checked by a D & C on an annual basis. So please talk to your doctor about this.

Q **I am now 53 and have not had a period for over eight months. Do I still need to use contraceptives?**

A No you do not. Once you are over 50 and have had six months without a period you are quite safe.

Q **Is osteoporosis really such a worry for women after the menopause?**

A Osteoporosis, or thinning of the bones, does occur in women after the menopause. For one in every three it may mean that she will suffer more fractures, particularly of the hips, wrists, and spine. Bones can be kept healthy by regular exercise and by ensuring an adequate intake of calcium in the diet.

4
Healthy birth control

The decision about whether, or when, to have a family is of primary importance for all women. With today's more efficient contraception women can plan their families and careers, and take far more control over their lives. However, these new and more accurate methods of birth control are not without some risks, and it may be many years yet before the perfect method of contraception is developed.

Contraception

The Pill

Q **I would love to go on the Pill, but I am worried that I will find it all too confusing. I have read my friend's instruction sheet and it does seem very complicated.**

A Reading other people's drug information is not the most straightforward way to find out what you need to know. The Pill is very simple to take and either your doctor or your local Family Planning Clinic will take the time to explain to you exactly what is involved, so do go along and ask.

Q **Is it true that taking the contraceptive pill can protect you from cancer of the ovary?**

A Yes, it is. Taking any variety of combined pill, even for a few months, can reduce the risk of ovarian cancer developing by some 40 per cent. The effect probably takes between five and ten years to become apparent but it persists for at least 15 years after Pill use is discontinued. Ovarian cancer is the sixth most common cancer contracted by women, so anything which reduces this toll is to be welcomed.

Q **At 42, am I too old to start using the Pill? My health is good, apart from the occasional headache.**

A There isn't a straightforward yes or no answer, it depends on your 'risk factors'. If you smoke, are overweight, have had any circulatory problems, have a high blood fat content, suffer from high blood pressure, get bad migraines, have diabetes, or even a family history of heart attacks, or have any combination of these factors, you would certainly not be an ideal candidate for the Pill. In addition, most doctors do not encourage women over the age of 40 to use this form of contraception, even if they have no health risks. However, you might find that the progesterone-only pill is suitable for you.

Q **Just after I started taking the Pill I began to get very severe headaches. They come on in the Pill-free week and I would like to know if I can do anything about them.**

A The headaches sound as though they are related to hormone withdrawal, particularly of the progestogen component. If so, these can be cured rapidly by changing to a brand with a different progestogen.

Q Because my sex life is very infrequent I do not have any regular form of contraception. Is there a 'morning after' pill I could take on the few occasions I need it?

A Post-coital contraception has been around for many years but is not suitable for anything other than an emergency situation such as rape, or totally unprotected and unplanned intercourse. The 'morning after' pills contain a dosage of hormones that is almost seven times higher than you would take in a normal contraceptive pill and this is not something to subject your body to unless you have absolutely no choice.

Q Is the 'morning after' pill just one single dose?

A No, it consists of four pills altogether. Two contraceptive pills containing 50 mcg of oestrogen are taken straight away and then a further two tablets 12 hours later. It is essential that the full course of tablets be taken exactly as prescribed.

Q Does the 'morning after' pill have to be taken within a certain time of intercourse for it to work?

A Yes, the pills must be started within 72 hours of the unprotected intercourse, and the sooner the better.

Q I cannot take the Pill because I have had two attacks of thrombosis in the past. Of course, I can't take the 'morning-after' pill either so is there anything else I can do?

A Yes indeed. An intra-uterine device fitted as soon as possible, but certainly within 72 hours will usually prevent implantation, just like the 'morning-after' pill. Do discuss this with your doctor.

Other methods of contraception

Q **I have read that the IUD (intra-uterine device) has been banned in the USA. Should I have mine removed?**

A They have not been banned in the USA but have disappeared because the manufacturers have had such huge damages awarded against them that they have decided they cannot afford to allow them to be sold in that country. There is absolutely no evidence at all that the risks of the IUD are any different now to what they were some ten years ago. Unless there are particular reasons for you to have yours removed — check with your doctor if you want reassurance — it should stay where it is.

Q **Is it true that a coil can get lost? I had one put in a few months ago but now I can't find the string.**

A It is not uncommon for the threads of the coil to disappear. Normally the thread lies in the cervical canal linking the coil, which is inside the womb itself, with the outside world of the vagina. When the coil is inserted the thread may be cut too short so that when it settles into the womb the thread disappears into the canal. Or the thread may have simply folded up on itself so that although it is still present you can't feel it. Of course, it is always possible that it has just fallen out without your realizing it. Ask your doctor or Family Planning Clinic to check for you.

Q I use a cap for contraception but do sometimes worry about it letting me down. Is there something else I could do to be certain this didn't happen?

A You should always use a spermicidal cream with your cap and you should ask your partner to use a condom. This will minimize the risk if it is essential that you avoid a pregnancy.

Q Can I just buy a diaphragm over the counter without going to a doctor?

A You can certainly buy them without a prescription, but it would be of no use to you without having seen a doctor. It is essential that you are properly measured so that your diaphragm is a good fit. If it is too large then it will be too uncomfortable to use and if too small it will not fit over the cervix during intercourse, which is worse than useless. Once you have been properly fitted you can always buy a spare diaphragm direct from the pharmacist.

Q I have been using a diaphragm for the last two years and wonder how often it should be replaced?

A If you check it each time after you have used it, to make sure there is no damage or tears in the rubber, then you should only need to have a check up once a year to make sure that it is still the right size for you.

Q I went on a crash diet and lost a lot of weight. Does this mean I should change my diaphragm?

A Yes indeed you should have your size checked. Factors that can affect the fit of a diaphragm are abortion, childbirth and any sudden gain or loss of more than 14 pounds in weight.

Q How soon before intercourse can a diaphragm be inserted?

A The deciding factor really is the life span of the spermicide that is used with it. That is normally only six to eight hours and so the diaphragm should not be inserted more than two hours before intercourse. If intercourse is repeated within that period then more spermicide should be inserted into the vagina, using an applicator. *Do not remove the diaphragm to do this.*

Q How long must I leave the diaphragm in place after intercourse?

A At least eight hours to be certain that the sperm are no longer active. You can then remove it, wash and dry it and store it away from light and heat.

Q Is it really essential to use a spermicidal cream with my diaphragm?

A A diaphragm used alone is far less effective in preventing conception than when used with a spermicidal agent. Sperm are extremely mobile and can swim round the edges of even the newest and best-fitting diaphragm. This is where the spermicide takes over.

Q I have been using a diaphragm for a few years and have had one or two 'near misses'. I am worried that if I do have an accident I will not know about it until I miss my period. Is there anything I can do myself at that time if I think I am pregnant?

A Self-administered abortifacients are not yet available. However, anti-progesterone tablets are being developed which will interrupt valid pregnancies after the first missed period. It may be several years before these are available.

Q **How long can you leave a contraceptive sponge in place before the spermicide in it is not effective?**

A You should not leave a sponge in place for more than 24 hours. It should also not be removed until at least six hours after intercourse.

Natural family planning

Q **Is there a method of family planning that is very natural? I don't want to put chemicals or rubber into my body.**

A Yes, there is a method of checking when you are ovulating by comparing the changes in your mucus secretions throughout the month. These will vary between white and pasty, or clear and watery. Normally, as the oestrogen levels in your body rise in preparation for ovulation the quantity of mucus gradually increases and becomes clearer and thinner. Just before ovulation, the mucus is perfectly clear and very 'elastic' to the touch. You will need to do some very close observation on yourself to use this method, and it cannot be guaranteed to be 100 per cent accurate.

Q **Is there any way of making the mucus method more reliable?**

A It can be used best by combining it with a temperature chart which can identify ovulation, and a calendar marker for estimating your safe period.

Q **I want to use the rhythm method of family planning and wondered how to calculate when is the safe period?**

A Conception is much more likely if intercourse takes place a fortnight before the next period is due. This is the time when the egg ripens in the ovaries and becomes available for fertilization by the sperm. However, you really need to keep track of your menstrual pattern for at least six months to gauge when your most fertile time will be. Even then, pregnancy can occur quite a way either side of this and so you can never be entirely sure using this method.

Q **Why do they recommend keeping a chart of your temperature when using the rhythm method?**

A Because there is often a sharp rise in temperature just before ovulation. You can then use this as a guide to avoid intercourse during that time. However, do remember it is not foolproof.

Q **How do I know when I ovulate?**

A Ovulation takes place approximately 14 days before your next period is due. If your periods are regular then this is easy to calculate, but if not there are several DIY ovulation tests that can be bought from the pharmacist. However these are quite expensive so you may want to keep a check yourself to see if you can spot any of the signs; your temperature may rise, there may be a sharp pain in the groin area, some women experience a slight spotting or discharge, the secretions in the vagina change in colour and texture and with practice you may be able to recognize this.

Q I am breastfeeding my year-old baby and have not been using any method of contraception as I have not had a period yet. I thought that this would prevent me getting pregnant but my sister says this is not true.

A Breastfeeding does temporarily delay ovulation, but it is no guarantee that you will not become pregnant. Ovulation occurs two weeks before you menstruate, therefore if you wait for this to happen before you start using contraception you could be two weeks too late.

Abortion

Q How soon can a pregnancy test be done?

A Normally a doctor or clinic would want you to wait at least two weeks after the date your period was due. However, there are home testing kits available from the chemist which you can use from one to five days after your due date. No test is 100 per cent accurate, though, and the earlier it is done then the greater the possibility that there may be some error. You should still go to see your doctor or clinic a week or so later and have the diagnosis confirmed.

Q I am just over seven weeks pregnant and am quite certain that I cannot go on with this pregnancy. What type of abortion will I be offered?

A In the first eight to nine weeks a simple suction technique is used. The neck of the womb is only dilated a little and most operations are done on an out-patient basis. Late terminations (after 13 to 14 weeks) may need a mini Caesarean section, often called a hysterotomy, or will need drugs given by a drip to induce a premature labour.

Q **Are there any medical complications after having an abortion?**

A It will depend on what method has been used for the termination, how far pregnant you were and whether any other operation was carried out at the same time. Physical complications can arise immediately after the operation or much later on. Immediate complications are mainly due to excessive bleeding and infection and are more common in the more advanced pregnancy. Late complications can include infertility as a result of infection, and damage to the cervix which only shows up when you plan your next pregnancy.

Q **Do I need to have any further visits to the doctor after I have had an abortion?**

A Physical care following a termination is much like that after pregnancy. A medical check-up is usually carried out six weeks after the operation. Your surgeon will discuss this with you.

Q **I had an abortion two years ago. If I ever get pregnant again, or have to go into hospital for an operation, will I have to tell the doctors about the abortion?**

A Yes, your doctor will need to know if you had a blood transfusion associated with your abortion and if you know your blood group. If you are rhesus negative they will need to know if you were given an Anti D injection at the time of your abortion. If you were not, then it is possible you may have developed antibodies and you will be tested for this.

Q I have three children and am now pregnant again. I want to have an abortion as we do not want to increase our family. Can I also be sterilized at the same time?

A When sterilization is carried out at the same time as an abortion it significantly increases the complication rate, both physically and emotionally. For this reason surgeons prefer not to do both operations together, but you should discuss this with your doctor as soon as possible.

5
Healthy childbearing

Making sure you are fit and healthy *before* planning a family is one of the best ways of ensuring a trouble-free pregnancy. Childbearing is a natural function, not an illness, and pre-planning and good preparation will make sure you, and your baby, get off to a good start.

Pre-conception

Q **Is there any particular sexual position that favours conception?**

A Any position where the woman's legs are higher than her pelvis is often suggested. After intercourse you should lie still and relax for about twenty minutes with a pillow under your bottom. Gravity then gives nature a helping hand by keeping the semen high in your vagina.

Q **What happens to my baby if I contract German Measles while pregnant?**

A If you have not been vaccinated and you contract German Measles in the first three months of your pregnancy then your child has a one in ten chance of being born deaf or having cataracts. This is entirely preventable if you have the vaccination before conceiving.

Q I am planning on starting my family soon but have never been vaccinated for German Measles because I hate having injections. Is this one really necessary?

A Yes, it is vital to ensure that you are immune from German Measles (rubella) before you start planning a family. Ask your doctor to give you a blood test to find this out, and if you are not immune then you need to have the vaccination immediately because you will need to wait for three months before conceiving.

Q My partner and I are anxious to give our baby the best start in life. Is there anything in particular we can do to help before I become pregnant?

A If you both give up smoking and drinking then those two things really can make a difference. Not only will they aid conception but will also assist in a healthy pregnancy.

Q I am anxious to start a family and have stopped taking the Pill. My doctor says I should wait three months before trying to get pregnant. Why should I?

A It is a safety precaution to ensure that all the synthetic hormones contained in the Pill are out of your system and that your ovaries have returned to a normal regular rhythm. There is also some evidence that vitamin and mineral levels in the blood are altered by taking oral contraceptives and it is important to allow these levels to return to normal before you become pregnant.

Q My mother has just developed Huntington's Chorea and I am concerned that I might also develop it, or pass it on to any child I might have. What are the chances?

A Huntington's Chorea is a fairly uncommon condition but it *is* an inherited disease and there is no cure available at the moment of writing. There is about a 50 per cent chance of your having it and also passing it on to your unborn child.

Q My husband has ankylosing spondylitis. I am concerned about whether this is hereditary?

A There does seem to be a tendency for this disorder of the spine to be inherited. A special blood factor has been identified in sufferers which strongly supports the idea of inherited susceptibility. Your doctor should be able to give you further information.

Q I caught a bad form of hepatitis when I lived abroad and, although fully recovered, the doctors tell me I still carry the disease. I want to have a family soon, but is there any chance that my baby could be affected by the hepatitis?

A There is a small risk that your baby might become infected from you and you should discuss this possibility with your doctor. It is also very important that you warn the doctors and nurses dealing with you that you are a hepatitis carrier so that they can take special precautions when taking blood tests, as they too could become infected.

Q I live next to a family who have a little girl with cystic fibrosis. When I get pregnant could being in contact with her pass the disease on to my baby?

A Cystic fibrosis is the most common genetically inherited disease and affects the mucus making apparatus. It is in no way contagious. It is impossible for you or your baby to get it from any kind of contact with a sufferer.

Q My husband's younger brother has cystic fibrosis. Is our baby likely to be affected?

A To be affected a child must get two genes for this condition, one from his mother and one from his father. It is possible that one person in every 20 carries these abnormal genes, but even if you and your husband both have them then there would only be a one in four chance that the baby would have cystic fibrosis. Unfortunately there is no way of identifying people who are carriers and the fact that his brother has the condition does not mean that your husband necessarily also carries it.

Q My first baby has cystic fibrosis. Is there any way of telling whether or not my next child will also be affected?

A Your doctor or clinic should be able to offer you a test during your pregnancy to ascertain whether or not the baby has cystic fibrosis.

Q My husband's brother was born with a hare lip and I am worried about whether this condition is hereditary.

A There is about a one in 1000 chance of a baby having a hare lip and it is slightly more common in families who have a history of other children with this condition. However, treatment for it today is excellent so please don't worry about it.

Q **My husband's family has a history of Tay-Sach's disease and our doctor has suggested genetic counselling, but I am not pregnant. Isn't this too soon?**

A If there is a family history of an inherited problem then it can be wise to investigate it *before* you become pregnant. Your doctor can refer you to a specialized genetic centre for investigation to see if you or your husband would pass on a 'genetic' disability such as Tay-Sach's disease or haemophilia. Chromosome studies are very time-consuming and delicate, and though their accuracy record is very good they are not infallible.

Q **We have put off starting our family because of our commitments, but now, at the age of 33, I am pregnant. I am thrilled as we have waited so long, but is it true that Down's Syndrome is more common in babies born to older women?**

A It is true that Down's Syndrome babies are more common whether either the mother or the father is in their very late thirties or older. However, pregnancies are so much less common in this age group that the majority of parents of Down's Syndrome children had them in their twenties and early thirties.

Q **Is there a special test I can have to check whether I am carrying a Down's Syndrome child?**

A There is a blood test you can have for alpha fetoprotein and this is routine in many obstetric units. It is not specifically related to Down's Syndrome, but it is raised in a variety of conditions — even sometimes with a completely normal pregnancy. However, it is a simple test and if it is abnormal your obstetrician will recommend further tests.

Fertility

Q **Is there a rough guide to how long you have to try for a baby before you think of getting help?**

A It is usually reckoned that a woman using no contraception, and having intercourse an average of two to three times a week, can expect to get pregnant within five months. If there is no pregnancy by the end of 18 months then there could be a problem and it would be worth going to see your doctor.

Q **I believe I am suffering from infertility. Is it more likely to be my fault than my partner's?**

A Infertility is not a disease, it is a symptom of a whole variety of conditions. Around half of infertility problems can be traced back to the woman, a third to the man, and the rest are due to minor disturbances in both which then combine to create a problem. There is no question of establishing fault, but only in finding the best way of solving the problem.

Q **I am worried that I have not been able to get pregnant, despite trying for the last year. I don't want to upset my husband so should I see the doctor on my own first?**

A Ideally you should both go together so that you can support each other and give the doctor the fullest possible picture of the situation.

Q My husband and I have been trying to start a family for the last year without any success. I am so depressed about it, and feel as if anyone can get pregnant except those who want to.

A Please don't be discouraged. It can be heartbreaking when you are trying, without success, to become pregnant — but you are not alone. It is estimated that one in every 10 couples has a problem in starting a family, so please don't give up yet. Have you talked to your doctor? If not then please go along so that you and your husband can have a thorough investigation to check that there is no simple physical reason preventing conception.

Q My partner and I have been trying for a baby for two years. We both have very busy jobs and I also have to travel a great deal. Is the stress of all this having an effect on my fertility?

A Stress certainly doesn't help, but the basic requirement for conception is to be with your partner at the right time of the month. You may have to change your lifestyle to have more relaxed time together if you are really serious about having a baby.

Q I have been told that my infertility is as a result of having an operation for fibroids when I was in my twenties. How did this make me infertile?

A It is not common for young women to have fibroids, but when they do it is possible that they may distort either the lining of the womb enough to cause a miscarriage, or kink the Fallopian tubes which carry the eggs. Although your fibroid was removed, the operation may have left some scars.

Q **I was diagnosed as having a cervical erosion two years ago. I have been trying for a baby for the last year and the specialist has said that my previous condition could be preventing my getting pregnant. How could this happen?**

A Cervical erosion can be a factor in infertility. The sperm need everything just right for their hazardous swim into the Fallopian tubes, but the erosion makes acid mucus which may impair their ability to swim at all. Simple treatment of your erosion may be all that is necessary.

Q **I have polycystic ovary disease (PCOD) and want to start a family next year. Will this affect me?**

A Enlarged first time PCOD sufferers often have difficulty in becoming pregnant because the egg ripening process is disturbed. The follicle containing the mature egg does not pop at the right time. This failure disturbs other control systems in the body.

Q **We have been trying to have a baby for several years. My doctor has now suggested we try GIFT. What exactly is this?**

A The initials stand for Gamete IntraFallopian Transfer. An egg recovered from inside your body is mixed with sperm and then transferred immediately to the inside of your Fallopian tube — at the end nearest to the womb. The baby created by this method is part of you and your husband if his sperm is used. This technique of fertilization is especially useful for those women who have a blockage near the ovaries while the rest of the Fallopian tube is normal.

Q **We want to start a family in the next year or so, but my husband has just had a bad attack of mumps. Will this make him infertile?**

A Adult men do suffer more than most from an attack of mumps. They may get orchitis (inflammation of the testes) which can be very uncomfortable, with pain and swelling of the scrotum. But, although none of this will have made him feel very good, contrary to popular opinion mumps hardly ever leads to infertility.

Q **When I talked to the gynaecologist about my infertility she said my notes showed I'd had salpingitis several years ago and that this could be a contributory factor. I don't remember ever being told I had this, so what exactly is it?**

A Your doctor may just have referred to it as a pelvic inflammatory infection and it happens when microbes are introduced into the body — usually via the vagina during intercourse. The infection can spread to include the uterus, Fallopian tubes and ovaries and would usually have been treated with simple pain relievers or antibiotics if the condition was persistent.

Q **I had a miscarriage several years ago and have not been able to get pregnant since. Shortly afterwards, I had a bout of infection and my doctor now says I may have had salpingitis and that this may be a cause of my infertility. How could this have happened?**

A The salpinges, or Fallopian tubes, have very delicate mechanisms which facilitate the transport of the egg to the womb and the sperm to the egg. These mechanisms are damaged by infection, the tube itself may even become blocked. The womb and Fallopian tubes are very vulnerable to infection after childbirth or miscarriage and with very few exceptions salpingitis occurs in sexually active women. The exceptions are infection from tuberculosis, and secondary inflammation owing to a severe bout of appendicitis or colitis.

Q **I believe that the symptoms of salpingitis are very similar to lots of other common ailments. What should I look for?**

A The symptoms are, unfortunately, very non-specific. They are very similar to the symptoms of a urinary infection, a mild bout of diarrhoea or stomach upset, or an early or mild appendicitis. The infection gives symptoms of nausea, mild fever and tenderness. The tenderness is situated just above the groin and is usually felt on both sides equally. There may be some vaginal discharge or irregular vaginal bleeding. It is always very important to have an accurate diagnosis of acute or chronic lower abdominal pain because of the effect salpingitis may have on your future fertility.

Q **When we went to the Infertility Clinic we were advised not to have intercourse too often. Surely the more often we make love the better the chances of conception?**

A The aim here is to keep your partner's sperm count as high as possible. If he ejaculates every day, twice a day, then his sperm count will be lowered. Intercourse every third day in the early and late parts of the cycle, with daily intercourse around the time of ovulation, will give you the best chance of conception.

Q **My husband has finally agreed to go to the Infertility Clinic with me but is concerned about what is involved.**

A Some 33 per cent of all infertility is caused by problems with sperm production and delivery, so it is obviously important that your husband is checked as well as yourself. He will be asked to produce a semen sample and there are three main features which the clinic will want to measure: the numbers, normality and mobility of the sperm. He will also have a physical examination of his penis and testes to make sure they are normal.

Q **Is there anything my partner can do to increase his fertility, without going to a clinic?**

A There are some self-help measures that he might like to try, but they are no substitute for the accurate information a clinic will be able to give him. Stopping smoking and giving up alcohol can both improve the quality and performance of the sperm; keeping the testes cool by wearing loose fitting clothing also encourages the production of sperm. Some doctors also recommend bathing the testes every day in cold water, but swimming in cool water may be a more acceptable substitute.

Q **We have had all the tests possible and have been told that my husband is infertile. I am desperate to have a child and want to find out how successful artificial insemination is.**

A AID or Artificial Insemination by Donor, has been technically very successful in a number of cases, but the emotional (and possibly legal) traumas can be very real. It is only suitable for a small proportion of infertile couples and you and your husband need to be very secure — both in yourselves and with each other — before you consider it. When you and your husband have discussed it thoroughly then go back and seek your doctor's advice.

Miscarriage

Q **I am confused about the way losing a baby is sometimes called miscarriage and sometimes abortion. What do both mean?**

A Medically, any pregnancy that ends before the 28th week of gestation is an *abortion*. Doctors increasingly use the lay term *miscarriage* to describe an unplanned event, but this is also called a *spontaneous abortion*. Where an abortion has been deliberately induced it is called a *medically induced abortion* and the operation is called *termination of pregnancy*.

Q **How common are miscarriages and can anything be done to prevent them?**

A Unhappily, they are quite common. Around one in 15 pregnant women need to see their doctor about a miscarriage. Generally when a miscarriage occurs no specific cause is found so it is difficult to advise on any particular precautions.

Q I had a miscarriage two months ago and my husband is keen to try for another child. I do not feel ready yet, and am very worried about the possibility of losing another baby.

A Miscarriages are much more common in the first than in any subsequent pregnancy and it can be a very frightening and painful experience. Most women take at least three months to recover enough to try for a second pregnancy and to overcome the depression and sense of loss that accompanies a miscarriage. The vast majority of subsequent pregnancies, however, are entirely successful. Do let your husband know how you feel so you can both agree on the best time to try again.

Q I recently had a miscarriage when I was just ten weeks pregnant. I am a very active woman and wonder if this had anything to do with it and whether I should take things easy next time.

A Routine activity and occupations can do nothing to produce a miscarriage. In fact we wouldn't need abortion clinics if all we had to do was exercise. Losing a pregnancy before 13 weeks is most often due to hormone problems, but it may also be a way for the body to reject abnormally formed babies. These abnormalities are most commonly due to imperfect chromosome patterns, but some 15 per cent of all first pregnancies miscarry spontaneously without any obvious reason. The next pregnancy usually goes ahead without any problems.

Q **I read in the paper recently that VDU users are more likely to have miscarriages than ordinary typists. Is this true?**

A Recent studies in the USA have shown an increase in miscarriage but there are a lot of possible reasons why this might be. The age of the woman, her previous experience of miscarriage, whether this is her first pregnancy or not — these are all factors which influence the miscarriage rate which may vary between VDU operators and other typists. A recent British study showed no difference between them. Your local Health and Safety Office should be able to give you guidelines on the safe use of VDU's.

Pregnancy tests and examinations

Q **Why do you have to take an early morning urine specimen for pregnancy tests?**

A The urine gets very concentrated at night so that an early morning specimen contains more of the hormones which the tests are trying to discover. These hormones are produced by the developing afterbirth which is bedding into the mother's womb to get nourishment for the new baby. That is why it is important that the specimen should be taken immediately on getting up.

Q **Is it possible for a pregnancy test to be positive even if you are not pregnant?**

A Yes, it is, though it is unusual. There are two reasons. The first is if you have had a very early spontaneous miscarriage; this happens in 15 per cent of all conceptions. These very sensitive tests will diagnose pregnancy early and then you will go on a week or so later to have a normal period. The second reason for a positive test is very very rare and occurs where the test is reflecting high levels of hormones which are being made from a very rare womb cancer called choriocarcinoma. Anyone who persistently has a positive test, and who is not obviously pregnant, should discuss the findings with her doctor as a matter of urgency.

Q **I have recently bought a home pregnancy testing kit so I can know as soon as possible if I am pregnant. Why do they suggest testing twice?**

A The new tests are so accurate that they can be used immediately a period is missed. However, although the test is accurate the certainty of a pregnancy continuing is not. Many pregnancies, perhaps as high as 10 per cent, fail to implant properly. Although your test can be positive immediately your period is missed, a retest two weeks later may give a negative result. This is why most tests advise that your wait until you are at least five to six weeks away from your last period. Even with this precaution it is important to remember that home tests have a failure rate of one in every 100.

Q **I am making my first visit to the antenatal clinic soon. What will they want to know?**

A You will be asked to give a brief history of your past illnesses and any operations to date, plus details of any previous babies or pregnancies you have had.

Q **What sort of checks are carried out at an antenatal clinic?**

A You first have a general examination, including heart, lungs and blood pressure. The doctor will examine your stomach to see if the growing womb can be felt yet and there will then be an internal examination, possibly including a cervical smear. Other important parts of the first examination are a blood test to check you haven't got anaemia and to find out your blood group. Usually you will also have your blood tested for German Measles, and if you aren't immune you will be vaccinated after the birth. As a final check a urine test is also carried out.

Q **In an internal examination, what is the doctor checking for?**

A Your obstetrician will have a full check list. First — is the womb growing as expected? Second — are the pelvic bones well shaped? Third — are there any other masses like fibroids or ovarian cysts present?

Q **As I have a full-time job I am concerned about getting time off to go to the antenatal clinic. How often will I have to go?**

A Check-up visits which include monitoring blood pressure, urine, weight and examining the abdomen will take place every month until you are seven months pregnant, then every two weeks. Then for the final four week run-up you will be seen every week.

Q **I am due to have an ultrasound scan in the new few weeks to check that all is well with my baby. Could you tell me if this procedure is at all dangerous?**

A Ultrasound is entirely safe. Sound waves are passed through your body and they bounce back from the baby, showing its outline, where the afterbirth is situated, exactly how mature your baby is — and of course it (usually) confirms that there is only one and not two. You need have no fears at all.

Q **What is an amniocentesis?**

A The amnion is the sac of water that surrounds the baby in its mother's womb. This sac is made by the baby itself as it develops; this means that cells in the fluid have exactly the same make-up as the baby itself. At amniocentesis a very fine needle is passed into the womb and a few drops of amniotic fluid drawn off. If a sample of this fluid is grown in the laboratory, the cells can be examined for their chromosomes and any abnormalities, like Down's Syndrome, can be detected early.

Q **I am 35 and expecting my first baby. I have been offered an amniocentesis test, but am not sure whether to have it done.**

A Amniocentesis is a screening test and from it many inherited abnormalities can be detected. You must decide: would you want a termination if an abnormality was detected? Also, are you prepared to take the slight, but real, risk of losing the baby that the investigation itself carries? Unless you answer 'yes' to both these questions then amniocentesis would not be advisable.

Q Is it necessary to have an amniocentesis? I am to have one shortly and am very worried.

A Because the purpose of the test is to check on the health of your baby (see previous question) you should only undertake it if you would wish to have the pregnancy terminated if there was any abnormality. If you would not contemplate a termination under any circumstances then you should not go ahead with the test.

Q Two years ago I had an abortion. My husband never knew about this and I am now expecting another baby. I am worried about whether the hospital has to know about the abortion, and if they will tell my husband.

A The hospital certainly needs to know your full medical history so they can discover exactly what treatment you had at the time and whether they need to carry out any additional tests. This is essential both for your health and your baby's. You must be honest and tell them about your abortion, but you can say that you do not wish any written record to be made on your notes or for your husband to be informed. They will then institute any investigations they need, and once they have a record of your blood state, no more need be said.

During pregnancy

Q I am a very active person who enjoys a lot of sports. Must I give them up now I'm pregnant?

A No, not unless your doctor says you must and that will depend on what kind of sport you mean. Regular exercise is usually encouraged unless it is very strenuous or carries the risk of some injury to you or the baby. Talk it over with your doctor first.

Q **My sister has been told she has an ectopic pregnancy. What exactly is this?**

A An ectopic pregnancy is one that starts to develop in the wrong place. In the normal course of events the fertilized egg passes from the Fallopian tube into the womb, but if there is any delay in reaching the womb then the fertilized egg will 'nest' in the lining of the tube. Obviously as the foetus begins to grow the tube is stretched too much and the pregnancy is doomed.

Q **I'm now three months pregnant and I have suffered morning sickness from the very beginning. Is there anything I can do to ease it?**

A Take heart, it will almost certainly soon be over. Morning sickness is much more common in a first pregnancy and usually stops soon after the first three months have passed. If you have some tea and toast in bed first thing in the morning it will give your stomach something to work on before you start the day. Get up slowly and in good time so that you don't have to rush to start work. Although there are many quite innocent preparations that your doctor can prescribe for you to use at this stage in your pregnancy, it really is best to manage without any medication if you possibly can.

Q **I have heard that ginger can help with morning sickness. Is this true?**

A It is often suggested for travel sickness and has helped many women with this particular type of nausea. You might like to try taking ginger powder, dissolved in hot water, or in capsules to see whether it can help you.

Q **Why do I get so much heartburn now I'm pregnant?**

A It's because digestive acid from the stomach is entering your oesophagus and irritating the delicate lining. Unfortunately it's your 'bump' which is causing this, because it fills up your tummy and pushes the contents upwards towards your chest. Your muscles are not strong enough to prevent the digestive acid from slipping upwards into your food tube (oesophagus).

Q **I have been having a lot of trouble sleeping since I became pregnant. Would it be all right to take the occasional sleeping pill?**

A You should *never* take any drugs during pregnancy without the express advice of your doctor. Most would be reluctant to prescribe a sedative for you unless it was essential, particularly during the first 14 weeks of your pregnancy or if you are near to delivery because of the effects it could have on the baby.

Q **Backache has been a constant problem throughout my pregnancy. Is there anything I can do to relieve it?**

A First make sure that you are not overweight, as this can make the problem worse. A simple exercise that can help relieve the pain is to get down on all fours and then gently arch your back upwards — rather like a cat — and let your head fall forward between your shoulders. When you return to the rest position do make sure that your back is straight and not hollowed or you will give yourself even more backache. Do this a few times until you feel the pain has lessened.

Q **I know I am not supposed to smoke when I am pregnant, but I get so anxious sometimes that only a cigarette calms me down. Surely it is better for me and the baby if I am calm, rather than worrying about the odd smoke?**

A Smoking interferes with the blood supply of the placenta: women who smoke heavily have smaller babies and these babies may have problems at birth. Anxiety certainly isn't good for the baby, but if you could find some other way of soothing your nerves you will certainly increase your chances of having a healthier baby.

Q **My pregnant sister now refuses to have even one glass of wine when she comes to dinner. I have said one won't make any difference but she disagrees. Who is right?**

A Almost every pregnant woman feels she must do everything possible to protect her unborn child, and giving up alcohol and tobacco are two of the most important things she can do. Your sister is right — alcohol can harm her baby. You are right — one glass of wine probably doesn't matter, but if anything did go wrong with the baby could you (or she) live with the knowledge that your own thoughtlessness may have caused it? Let your sister make her own decisions, and support her to the full.

Q **I am eight months pregnant and seem to be putting on a lot more weight than I thought I would. Is there a rough guide to how much I should weigh?**

A Generally you would look to gain less than two stone (28 pounds/15 kilograms) during your pregnancy. It is important to keep within these limits as too much weight gained can be harmful for the baby — and difficult for you to lose after the birth.

Q **I am not sure about whether to breastfeed my baby. My mother says that if I do the baby will be protected against stomach upsets. Is this true?**

A Breast milk does contain antibodies that help protect your baby against the many harmful germs that are encountered once outside the protective conditions of the womb. When a small baby comes across a germ s/he cannot handle, this sets up an inflammation of the stomach and intestines — gastroenteritis. This infection causes the gut to push the food through before any of its goodness has been digested, and most importantly, before the water has been absorbed. This can lead to dehydration. Gastroenteritis in babies should always be reported to a doctor as the child can so rapidly become very ill.

Q **I am expecting twins shortly and at my last check up I heard the doctor say I had a minor case of hydramnios. What is this exactly?**

A It means that there is an extra amount of amniotic fluid surrounding the babies, and this does seem to be more common when there are twins. In a minor case all that is required is to take more rest.

Q **I have never been keen on any form of keeping fit and now the midwife keeps trying to give me exercises to do after the baby is born. Is this really necessary?**

A Yes! After pregnancy it is vital that the pelvic muscles are exercised back into shape. They support the womb, the bladder and the rectum and if the pelvic floor is not fully restored after birth then prolapse of the womb can occur in later life. This can generally be avoided by exercise and early mobilization after childbirth, so try and look on it as a good preventative measure, not a chore.

Q **At a recent antenatal check-up the doctor said my baby was 'small for dates'. What did he mean exactly?**

A It is a title used to describe any baby who does not grow at the expected rate while still in the womb. There are several ways of measuring such growth. The very simplest is just to measure how big the womb is at various stages of pregnancy. At 14 weeks from the date of the last period the womb can usually just be felt in the stomach, at 24 weeks it has reached the navel and at 36 weeks it is usually at its biggest and reaches the rib cage. Ultrasound testing is much more accurate at measuring the baby's size and this can then be plotted against tables showing expected size at a particular stage.

Q **Are there any particular factors which govern a baby's weight and size?**

A The size of the mother is important — small people have small babies. It is unusual for Indian women, for example, to have babies that weigh more than eight pounds. Medical conditions are also important. Raised blood pressure in the mother which is causing placental problems can limit the nutrition of the baby, causing quite important growth retardation. That is why it is so important to visit the antenatal clinic for regular blood pressure checks. Women who smoke tend to have smaller babies and of course if you are having twins or triplets then they tend to have smaller weights than a single baby would. However, size is not necessarily connected to health and most small babies go on to become very healthy adults.

Q **What is the normal blood pressure during pregnancy?**

A It is not possible to give figures because each woman is slightly different, and as the pregnancy goes on the blood pressure will change. From it's 'normal' rate at the beginning it usually falls around the fourth month and then rises again towards the birth. It is important that you have it checked regularly throughout your pregnancy; every month at the beginning and weekly by the end.

Q **I am expecting twins but want to carry on much as normal. Is there really much difference between carrying one baby and carrying two?**

A Because of the extra volume of baby, water and afterbirth that you will be carrying the actual mechanics of a twin pregnancy may force you to take life much more easily. You need to put your feet up more and bending and stooping can be almost impossible. There is also the extra chance of developing high blood pressure, which again will require more rest.

Q **My husband and I are planning to go to a family wedding which is over 100 miles from our home. The problem is that it is only six weeks before our babies are due — we are having twins — and I am not sure if I should travel.**

A Twins are often born earlier than expected. The womb is stretched as far as possible and because of this it can decide earlier than usual that it has had enough and go into labour. Long-distance travel, indeed any kind of away-from-home visits, are not a good idea in the last six weeks before the expected birth date of twins.

Q **I have just been told that I am expecting twins and I don't know where to go for advice.**

A The best advice usually comes from someone in the same situation, so ask your doctor or clinic if they can put you in touch with any mothers who have had twins recently.

Q **I have been getting a heavy discharge for the last two weeks. It is quite clear and I am worried in case it is my waters leaking. I am in the last month of my pregnancy.**

A A lot of clear mucus is normal in pregnancy. If it is water than it can be leakage from either your bladder or the womb. Smell the discharge, if it is urine then this is again quite common in pregnancy, but if it is water you should tell your doctor so they can test if it is leaking from the womb.

Q **How long can I carry on working before the baby is born?**

A It can vary according to what kind of job you have. The 28th week of pregnancy is when many women stop, but provided you feel well then there is no reason why you can't work until a week or so before the baby is born.

Sex and pregnancy

Q **Now that I am pregnant I find my 'bump' gets in the way when making love. What would be a good position?**

A Being comfortable is very important, so try making love side by side, on top of your partner or let him approach you from behind.

Q I am 16 weeks pregnant. My husband still wants to make love but I am worried in case it hurts the baby. Could you tell me whether there is a chance this could happen?

A Lovemaking is entirely normal throughout pregnancy when it is comfortable for both partners, and will neither cause abortion nor hurt the baby. However, there are two situations when it should be avoided. The first is if a woman has previously had a miscarriage in the first 13 weeks of pregnancy, then it might be wise to avoid sex during that same period in a new pregnancy. The second is after the waters have broken, particularly when this happens some time before labour starts.

Q Since I've become pregnant my husband doesn't want to make love at all. I have made a few overtures but he has not responded. I still want to have a sex life, so why is he behaving like this?

A Men can be afraid of harming the baby through sex, so you will just have to explain to him that there is no contact between him and the baby during intercourse. If he is still worried, then mutual masturbation might help relieve some of your frustration.

Q How soon after the birth can I start making love with my partner?

A As soon as you feel ready for it, provided the birth has been a straightforward one. You vagina will probably be fairly tender for at least ten days after the birth and if you had an episiotomy this tenderness may continue for longer.

Q My baby was born six weeks ago and I am still tender when my husband makes loves to me. Is this usual or is something wrong?

A Any vaginal pain that persists after the six week check-up should be referred to a doctor. It is possible that one of your stitches has not properly dissolved or there is still an area of raw skin in the vagina itself. Either way your doctor can treat you for this discomfort.

Problems that can occur

Q I am in the last stages of pregnancy and the lips of my vagina have become blue and swollen. What is causing this?

A Some swelling of the lips of the vagina is very common, due to poor circulation. You may also have a few varicose veins of the vulva, which is the area around the vagina. If this problem does not clear up after the birth you should ask your doctor for help.

Q My mother has warned me that now I am pregnant I must be careful to avoid piles. Why should I be prone to them?

A It is a common condition in pregnancy because the stomach is stretched and presses on the veins around the back passage and this can start off piles — also known as haemorrhoids. It can be worse after the birth itself when the thought of passing a motion with the (unfounded) fear of possibly bursting the stitches makes a visit to the lavatory a very tense affair. The best way to avoid them is to keep to a sensible diet and regular habits so that you avoid constipation and overstraining.

Q **How can I alleviate the discomfort of varicose veins around the vagina?**

A It will help if you put a pad inside your pants to apply pressure to the area. Put it on after lying down for a short while with your bottom raised on a pillow. A fairly firm pair of pants may be needed to keep it on. While you are lying down it might help to make an ice pack to put against the sore area. Put some icechips in a small polythene bag, wrap a clean cloth around it and apply to the swollen parts. Be careful not to put your weight on it because it can cause damage to the delicate tissue if pressed hard against your flesh.

Q **Why should I be more prone to varicose veins just because I am pregnant?**

A Pregnancy is a real risk factor because as the womb enlarges it presses on the major veins in the abdomen. This can obstruct the flow of blood from the feet. You can help prevent varicose veins developing by observing the frequent advice given to pregnant women; 'never stand when you can sit, never sit when you can lie down'.

Q **After the birth of my first child I was left with a flabby piece of skin just inside the vagina. This has never disappeared and recently a small lump formed just underneath the skin. I am now pregnant again and this lump has got larger and has a white head on it. It doesn't hurt or itch but I am worried in case it might affect the baby in some way.**

A It sounds like an ordinary whitehead, or a small sebacious cyst. There has probably been an infection of the hair follicles or a blockage of the sweat glands, but there is no cause for alarm at all. Just show the lump to the doctor on your next antenatal check up.

Q   **At the antenatal clinic I heard the doctor talking about one of the patients having PET. What is this?**

A   It is an abbreviation for Pre-Eclampsia Toxaemia which is a serious disease that normally only occurs in the later stages of pregnancy. One of the reasons that antenatal check-ups are so important is so that conditions like PET can be identified. One of the earliest signs of PET is a raised blood pressure and this is checked at each antenatal clinic visit. PET is harmful in two ways; first it reduces the blood supply providing nutrition so that the baby fails to grow properly. Such a baby is very much under stress at the time of birth and for the first few days of its life. Also, if PET is left unchecked, it can harm the mother by causing eclamptic fits which are rather like epileptic fits and can threaten the life of mother and baby.

Q   **What are the symptoms of PET?**

A   The first sign is usually a rise in blood pressure, and there can also be swollen ankles and sometimes signs of kidney damage which show up as a protein deposit in the urine.

Q   **What is the treatment for PET?**

A   The bodily changes that are associated with PET can vary enormously in severity and if you are having regular antenatal checks then it is rare for a case to be far advanced. Treatment is usually lots of rest, in hospital if the case is severe, with perhaps some medication to bring the blood pressure down.

Childbirth

Q Is it possible to have a painless childbirth?

A A few women do experience a painless childbirth. The majority, however, do feel some pain — especially at the first birth. Relief is offered by the maternity staff in the form of pethidine, gas and oxygen, or epidural analgesia. In most cases this goes a long way towards making the pain entirely tolerable.

Q What is an epidural?

A It's where an anaesthetic is injected into the base of your spine during labour to temporarily numb the nerves that cover the lower half of your body.

Q Why is it so important to go to antenatal relaxation classes?

A At antenatal relaxation classes you will learn how to relax, how to manage your breathing, and a good approach to the coming birth. This will help you, your baby, and the labour ward staff.

Q How will I know when the baby is ready to be born?

A You will start to get contractions, irregularly at first then in an increasing tempo as the birth gets nearer. There is also a 'show' of a blood-stained discharge and when labour is quite near the membranes rupture and there is a leakage of amniotic fluid, either slowly or in a sudden rush.

Q **Do I have to have an enema before the birth?**

A It is preferable to have an empty bowel before you give birth, but this can be achieved without an enema.

Q **How long does labour usually last?**

A It is very difficult to say because no two women are alike. But, generally speaking, the first stage of labour (from when contractions start up to the full dilation of the uterus) takes less than 24 hours for a first baby, and six to eight hours for subsequent births. However, it can take much less, or more time depending on the individual concerned. The second stage, when the contractions become much more powerful and the baby is pushed out of the birth canal, is much shorter. This can be up to two hours for a first baby, and perhaps 30 minutes for subsequent births. Finally, the placenta is expelled and this is usually around 15 minutes after the baby has been born, though it can take as long as an hour.

Q **What is a breech birth?**

A When the baby comes down the birth canal bottom first instead of the more normal head first.

Q **If my baby is very overdue will it have to be induced?**

A Induction is only carried out when the doctor believes that to allow the pregnancy to go on presents a threat to the health of the mother or the child.

Q **How is the birth induced?**

A The doctor examines you to see whether your cervix is ready to begin labour. If it is not, then a special pessary will be inserted into the vagina. This will cause the uterus to contract and the cervix to open. A cut is then made into the membranes surrounding the baby to allow the amniotic fluid to filter out. If these measures do not work then a synthetic hormone is given by intravenous drip. The purpose of this is to further encourage the uterus to contract and allow labour to begin.

Q **I am frightened that I might have to have a forceps delivery. Surely this must hurt the baby?**

A Forceps are only ever used to *help* a baby, not to harm it. The forceps are specially shaped so that they cannot press unduly onto a baby's head or hurt it in any way.

Q **What is an episiotomy?**

A It is a cut about one to one-and-a-half inches long which is made from the vagina towards the back, and a bit towards the side. It is made to assist the baby to come out easily. An injection of local anaesthetic is usually given first to numb the area.

Q **I am afraid of having an episiotomy. Is it really essential?**

A If you really do not want to have one then you must ask to have your notes marked with your preference 'does not want episiotomy' and be sure to remind the hospital staff at the time of the birth. However, do remember you may tear the skin anyway. This will require stitches, and can be much larger and take longer to heal properly than a planned episiotomy.

Q **Why is an episiotomy carried out?**

A Although generally the doctor will try to deliver the baby without making a cut, s/he may want to hurry the birth along. For example, if the baby's heartbeat is slow and s/he is are concerned about a shortage of oxygen. Having an episiotomy also helps to prevent excess stretching of your muscles and may prevent you having a prolapse later.

Caesarean

Q **What are the sort of problems that make a surgeon decide to perform a Caesarean?**

A The reasons may be related to the size or presentation of the baby, the birth canal or to problems with the afterbirth. Most of the Caesareans in the first pregnancy will be done as a result of some problem arising either in late pregnancy or during labour. A planned Caesarean section is not common in a first pregnancy unless the mother has very high blood pressure which refuses to respond to treatment, or the baby is coming breech first.

Q **If I have a Caesarean does this mean I won't be awake to see my baby being born?**

A While most women do have a general anaesthetic for their Caesarean, a spinal or epidural anaesthetic is quite common. If you have this, you are awake and can watch the baby being born — although you feel no pain — and even hold him or her while the surgeon stitches up.

Q **I had my first baby by Caesarean. Does this mean I can't give birth normally next time?**

A No, not necessarily, it depends on the reason for the first one. However, once you have had two Caesareans then almost all obstetricians would advise you that the operation will be necessary for all future births.

Q **If I have a Caesarean will there be much of a scar?**

A The surgical cut may either be from the navel downwards, or from side to side just above the hair line. This depends very much on the surgeon's choice but you can certainly express your preference. Whichever way, it usually heals rapidly and normally leaves only a small scar.

After the birth

Q **I have heard that you can get puerperal fever after childbirth but am not sure exactly what it is.**

A Puerperal fever is an infection of the genital tract and usually occurs within two weeks of the birth. It is marked by a high temperature and is treated with antibiotics. The widespread use of both antiseptics and antibiotics has meant that this is now a very rare condition.

Q **I had been warned about post-natal depression, but it still took me by surprise. How common is it?**

A Up to four out of every five mothers, particularly of first babies, get some degree of 'baby blues'. Really serious depression which goes on for some weeks or months affects around two in every 1000 new mothers. It has even been known to occur in women who have adopted a new baby.

Q **I never had any problems when my baby was born, I was just delighted with her. But now, a few weeks later I feel isolated and quite violent towards her. What is the matter with me?**

A Although you may not have had any symptoms just after the birth, you are now suffering from depression and this is often associated with aggression towards the baby. Your doctor and health visitor can help a great deal and you need to talk about it with them as a matter of urgency.

Q **What causes post-natal depression?**

A One theory is that it is due to the sudden drop in the circulation of progesterone, which is made in large quantities in the placenta. When the placenta is expelled from the body the production of the hormone is suddenly stopped and does not restart until menstruation is re-established. Another factor is the stress involved in adjusting to this major life change. Tiredness and sheer physical fatigue play a large part too.

Q Since having my baby daughter last year, I have had a post-natal examination and smear test. The results were satisfactory. However, while using tampons during my periods I can feel a small blob, that's the only way to describe it. As the doctor didn't seem concerned I have been reluctant to bother him again.

A It is most likely that you can feel your cervix (neck of the womb). To touch, it should feel rather like the end of your nose. Pregnancy can cause the pelvic floor to drop a little and it would be wise anyway to do some exercise to keep this firm and to avoid problems like prolapse.

Q Since my baby was born recently, I just don't feel hungry. I went off food during my pregnancy and now I am losing weight even though my child is now 18 months old. I just can't seem to put on weight. Why is this?

A It seems that your net energy loss is greater than your food intake. You are probably rushing around more and are not allowing yourself proper time for the food that you need. Perhaps you also need to rest more — difficult with a toddler, but see if others can help you out. Do go to see your doctor for a proper check-up to make sure that this is purely an eating problem, and nothing else.

Q In hospital they gave me salt water baths after my baby was born. What was the purpose of them?

A Salt water baths have a long history of healing because salt stops certain virulent bacteria from growing. So soaking in it can help eliminate any infection. They are often prescribed after episiotomies and the tears that occur naturally in childbirth. But bathing without the salt is probably just as beneficial.

Q **I gave birth a few weeks ago and have just noticed some stretch marks on my stomach. I had a good pregnancy and ate all the right foods. Why has this happened?**

A It is entirely normal to notice stretch marks after the baby is born and when your abdomen is so much smaller than before. Stretch marks are due to scars in the elastic tissue in the depth of the skin. They seem to run in families and be an inherited characteristic of the type of skin you have. So it doesn't make much difference what you do in terms of diet and exercise as you are unlikely to be able to prevent them.

Q **When my daughter was born the hospital said she was premature. Although she only weighed 4lbs 8oz she was born at the time that she was expected so I don't know what they meant.**

A There are two categories of premature babies. True premature babies are those born well before 40 weeks of normal gestation. Then there are a second group who are born at about the right time but don't achieve full growth in the womb. In the UK all babies who weigh less than 5lb 8oz (2.5kg) at birth are labelled as premature. It is just a guideline to identify a group of children who may be particularly at risk, both in labour and just after they are born. Like all guidelines it has flaws, small parents often have small children who are perfectly mature and are at no special risk — they just weigh less than 5lb 8oz.

Breastfeeding

Q My breasts became very hard and sore just after my baby was born. Why was this?

A A few days after your baby was born the milk supply began. This happens so swiftly that the breasts swell up and become hard and sore. This is called engorgement. It can also happen to women who stop breastfeeding, or whose baby has missed a feed.

Q What can I do about the discomfort of engorged breasts?

A The simplest thing to do is to feed your baby. Bathing your breasts in hot water will have the effect of softening them and you should always wear a good support bra night and day. If the discomfort is severe, then take some analgesics for the pain. When you stop feeding, use a bra until the milk has quite dried up.

Q How will engorgement affect my baby's feeding?

A Because the nipple is so swollen, your baby may not be able to suckle easily. If you express some of the excess milk from the breast first it will make it easier for you. You can express very gently by hand or use a breast pump.

Q I would like to breastfeed but am worried about losing my figure.

A That doesn't happen. In fact breastfeeding helps to use up fat stores in the body and so helps you keep your figure, not lose it.

Q   **I seem to have a hard lump in my right breast. It isn't affecting my breastfeeding, but what is causing it?**

A   It's possible you may have a blocked milk duct, but if it does not disappear after you massage the breast and bathe it in hot water then see your doctor straight away. It is always possible to get other breast problems, even when you're breastfeeding.

Q   **I have a breast abscess and my doctor has prescribed antibiotics. Is it alright to carry on breastfeeding?**

A   In general, yes, though do check with your doctor. There is usually no problem with continuing to feed your baby while being treated for the infection.

Q   **Can I do anything to prevent my nipples becoming cracked when I'm breastfeeding?**

A   Prevention is always better than cure, so start before the baby is born by 'toughening up' your nipples. In the last couple of weeks of your pregnancy, rub the nipples gently on a towel each time you wash and try leaving your bra off for a short time each day.

Q   **The doctor said that the abscess in my breast was caused by the fact that my nipples were cracked. What can I do about it?**

A   Cracked nipples are quite common after childbirth and it is then relatively easy for infection to enter through the crack and cause abscesses. The best method of protection against them is to look after the nipples by drying them thoroughly after each feed and to check that the baby is not causing any problems by dragging on the end of the nipple instead of taking the whole of it into the mouth.

Q **My sister, who is a nurse, has told me not to wash my nipples with soap while I'm pregnant. What is the reason for that?**

A The nipples contain natural oils which protect them, but soap will dry these out and leave you more prone to cracking and soreness.

Q **When feeding my baby I get a sharp pain in my left nipple. What is causing this?**

A You may have a thin crack in the nipple, so do ask your doctor or nurse to check it for you. S/he will give you a soothing cream which should heal it in a few days and will tell you how best to manage the crack. If you stop feeding your breast may become very tender, so you must express the milk.

Q **Can I do anything to stop my breasts becoming droopy after I have had the baby?**

A Make sure you wear a good support bra in your pregnancy and during lactation. This makes sure that the ligaments which anchor your breasts to the chest wall do not become stretched and helps maintain your shape.

Q **I am feeding my baby myself, and to my surprise my periods have started again as normal. I thought breastfeeding stopped all that?**

A After having a baby, the length of time before you start menstruating again can vary enormously. Breastfeeding does delay periods starting and they *may* not come back until feeding stops. But it is also quite normal for the periods to recommence during the time you are breastfeeding.

6
A healthy body and a healthy mind

Heart, circulation and respiratory system

Heart

The heart is a large muscle which works as a pump to send blood to all parts of the body. The output of blood from the heart is about three to five litres a minute during normal activity, but can rise to as much as ten litres per minute as a response to exertion of any kind. Having a healthy heart is something that can be worked on through sensible diet, exercise and avoiding being overweight or smoking or drinking too much.

 Is it true that stress can cause heart disease?

The simple answer is that no one knows. There are a group of people who react badly to stress and they do seem to be slightly more prone to heart disease than the rest of the population. However, stress cannot be blamed for the majority of heart problems because there are so many other factors to take into account.

Q **What is meant by high blood pressure and what causes it?**

A Everyone's blood pressure varies minute by minute, day by day. Strenuous exercise, anxiety or stress will all cause your blood pressure to rise because your heart is having to pump harder to move the blood around your body. This kind of increase will drop as soon as you relax or stop exercising.

Q **Why does blood pressure go up when you get hardening of the arteries?**

A Blood pressure will rise as the arteries become narrowed; the heart has to pump even harder to force the blood through the narrowed opening. This kind of increased blood pressure does not go down with rest but will require active management to get it back to a normal level.

Q **I have been treated recently for hardening of the arteries. On my last visit to the health centre I saw a new doctor. She asked if I was seeing a chiropodist regularly. What on earth have my feet to do with my heart condition?**

A If you suffer from any condition which reduces the blood circulation to your feet, such as hardening of the arteries or diabetes, then it is important to have your feet regularly checked. When circulation to that area is poor then the risk of infection getting in through a blister or any kind of cut to the skin is very great indeed. If this happens then the resulting infection can be very troublesome. Your doctor was just making sure you were taking preventative measures to avoid this.

Q If I have high blood pressure can I do anything about it?

A Yes, this is an area where you can do a great deal to help yourself before you have to resort to medication. Make sure that you are not overweight, give up smoking, and gradually increase the amount of exercise you take.

Q What should I do about my diet if I have high blood pressure?

A Take a careful look at exactly what you eat. Cut out added salt, reduce the amount of fat and sugar, and increase the fibre content by eating more fresh fruit and vegetables.

Q Would yoga help with my high blood pressure?

A It certainly does seem to help a lot of people control their blood pressure and can be used to relieve the stress and anxiety that often accompanies this condition.

Q My mother has had high blood pressure for a few months now and seems to have taken it well in her stride. What effect does it have on her system?

A High blood pressure can damage the walls of the blood vessels which have to withstand it. The muscles round the blood vessels get tighter in response to high blood pressure and this itself can increase the resistance and make the heart pump harder — this increases the blood pressure and the vicious cycle starts again.

Q **I know all about the dangers of high blood pressure, but I have *low* blood pressure. Does this mean I can never suffer a heart attack?**

A Low blood pressure is a good thing to have if it is your regular normal level. People with low blood pressure are generally less likely to have a heart attack than those with high blood pressure — but of course this cannot be guaranteed to be the case for everyone.

Q **If I stand up too quickly I get quite dizzy. What makes this happen?**

A Some people with low blood pressure also have blood vessels which are sluggish in responding to changes of position. This is probably what is happening to you. When you stand up suddenly, for instance, it makes you giddy. If this is a new experience for you it should always be checked out by a doctor.

Q **What causes a heart attack?**

A A heart attack is caused by a sudden cut off in the blood supply to the heart. In turn, this is often caused by a build-up of fatty deposits in the arteries which gradually causes them to narrow. This restricts the flow of blood to the heart. Spasm of the coronary arteries can also cause blockage. If the spasm does not ease, or if there is not a good bypass system, then a heart attack will occur.

Q There is quite a history of heart attacks in my family but all on the male side. I am concerned about whether I could have inherited this tendency too?

A If any member of your family has had a heart attack then it is obviously sensible to keep an eye on your own health. Men do run a greater risk of heart attacks but women are not immune. You could ask your doctor to carry out a blood test to see if you have inherited high blood cholesterol from your parents.

Q I know I have high blood cholesterol and wondered if my children could be tested to see if they also have it?

A Yes they can, in fact the test can be carried out on children over a year old. However, it's not very valuable until your children are in their teens, as most children have very low cholesterol levels.

Q Are there any foods which raise cholesterol levels?

A The saturated fats found in dairy products, meat and eggs tend to raise cholesterol levels and should be eaten in moderation, if at all, if you suffer from high blood cholesterol.

Q I have read that taking an aspirin a day can prevent heart attacks. If this is true shouldn't we all be taking them?

A Taking an aspirin a day is very worthwhile for people who have *already had* one heart attack. It is a simple precaution that might help to prevent another. It also seems to be useful for people who have suffered transient ischaemic attacks or minor strokes. A word of caution is necessary: the aspirin should only be taken after checking with your own doctor.

Q **Are there any special conditions attached to taking aspirin to prevent heart attacks?**

A Yes, aspirin should *never* be taken at the same time as taking anticoagulants, or if you have any history of peptic ulcers.

Q **If I take aspirin daily to prevent a heart attack, how do I take it?**

A It is always best to take aspirin in a soluble form and with food. Never on an empty stomach.

Q **When my mother died the death certificate said myocardial infarction. What does it mean?**

A It is the medical term for a heart attack.

Q **Since my father died two years ago of a heart attack I run the family business alone. I smoke more now than I used to and am worried that I am more at risk from a heart attack myself now.**

A The fact that your family has a history of heart disease is certainly an important factor, as is the increased stress and workload that you have taken on. People who smoke are more likely to suffer a heart attack than those who don't. So whilst you can't change what happened to your father, you can change the other risks in your life that are within your control.

Q **Are heart attacks always fatal?**

A No, only about a third of heart attacks are fatal immediately and the most dangerous time seems to be within the first two to three hours of the first attack.

Q **I am waiting to have a pacemaker fitted and wondered if you could explain exactly what it is and how it works?**

A Pacemakers were developed to take over and set a heart rate when the normal pacemaker in the heart fails. A very fine wire is threaded down a main vein until the tip is touching the inside of the heart wall. This wire is connected to a small electric battery which discharges an impulse regularly. This impulse takes over from the faulty mechanism.

Q **Where do the batteries go for a pacemaker?**

A The battery can be worn outside the body, on a belt for instance, if the pacemaker is only being used temporarily during the period of recovery from a heart attack. If it is needed permanently then the battery is usually implanted under the skin of the chest wall so that there is no danger of it being damaged or disconnected.

Circulation

Q **What exactly is angina?**

A It is a pain in the chest, usually brought on by exertion, and is caused by an insufficient blood supply to the heart — usually because the arteries are narrowed. The symptoms are a gripping or crushing pain which varies in severity from an unpleasant sensation to severe anguish.

Q **What causes angina pains to come on?**

A The pain is the result of the heart muscle being asked to work too hard. It is brought on by any exercise or exertion which increases the heart rate beyond a certain point.

Q **I have had angina for some time now, but the pain seems to get worse not better. What's the reason for this?**

A When a person first suffers from angina they can often carry out a lot of exercise before the pain starts, but gradually the pain commences after diminishing levels of exercise. Anger and rage can also bring on angina as they put up the pulse rate. Stopping the exercise, or calming down from your temper, will let the heart return to its normal rate and the pain will stop.

Q **The doctor referred to my mother's angina as a warning. But a warning of what?**

A A warning that the heart cannot cope. This is because the blood vessels feeding it are filled up with fatty deposits, known as atheroma, and this reduces the blood which is able to pump through them. These deposits never go away of their own accord but there are a number of ways of improving the situation.

Q **How is angina treated?**

A There are two ways you may be treated. Firstly there are drugs which will be prescribed to remove the pain of angina and to prevent attacks by dilating the blood vessels to the heart. However they do not remove its cause — the poor blood supply. Secondly, there is surgery and there are two options which can be very effective; coronary artery bypass and angioplasty.

Q **What is angioplasty?**

A Angioplasty is a much newer technique than a coronary bypass. A tiny tube with a deflated balloon at the end is passed right into the damaged coronary artery. The balloon is then inflated to crush the obstruction. The tube is removed from the heart and the blood flow is restored.

Q **What can I do myself to help my angina?**

A It is very important that you do what you can to help yourself. It will make a great difference to your progress. You must improve your physical fitness as much as you are able, give up smoking and make sure you are not even a couple of pounds overweight.

Q **What is coronary heart disease?**

A It is the name given to the narrowing of the coronary arteries which carry blood to the heart muscle and enable it to function properly.

Q **What does a coronary bypass involve?**

A Small veins are removed from the leg and used to bypass the blocked up stretch of coronary arteries which are supplying — or rather, not supplying — the heart muscle. The original blocked artery remains in place.

Q **My mother has had unsightly varicose veins for years. What causes them?**

A Varicose simply means distended and is really just a descriptive word, not a diagnosis. Veins are thin walled tubes and all along their length there are valves which ensure that the blood keeps moving towards the heart. Two main problems can cause the system to break down; anything which puts increased pressure on the abdomen (such as in pregnancy or being overweight), or a weakness in the valve system which allows the blood to stretch the vein walls.

Q **What can I do to help prevent varicose veins developing?**

A It is important to do everything you can to help keep your veins in good condition. Get plenty of exercise and keep your weight down. If you have to stand for long periods then try to make sure you don't stand *still*. Shift the weight from one leg to the other so that the leg muscles are kept moving. Making the muscles work will reduce the pressure on your veins and may help you avoid getting varicose veins.

Q **What treatment is there for varicose veins? I have a large vein on the front of my leg which is very obvious but I don't want to go into hospital for a long stay.**

A Established varicose veins can be difficult to treat, but if you simply have a few ugly-looking veins it may be possible to treat them by injection and this is almost always an out-patient procedure. If the vein needs surgical removal by stripping then this needs a general anaesthetic and can be done as a day case or may need an overnight stay in hospital.

Q I have quite a few varicose veins in my legs but they are not really very painful, just unsightly. What treatment is there for them?

A If they do not bother you then there is no need to have them treated. Support hosiery may be all that you will need, but if they do get worse then there are two options, injection or operation.

Q I am going to have a large and ugly varicose vein injected soon. Can you tell me exactly how this will make the vein look better?

A Injections involve a special chemical which cause the veins to collapse and vein walls to stick together. The injected vein becomes obliterated and eventually disappears.

Q My mother is having surgery for her varicose veins. What will the surgeon do?

A In surgery the veins are either tied off in several places, or the whole dilated vein can be stripped out.

Q Once I have had my varicose veins treated can they recur?

A Not those same veins, no, because they will have either been operated on or injected. However, whichever treatment you have it is obvious that the blood still has to travel somewhere; it will go through other veins and it is possible that they too may become varicose in time.

Q My mother and sister both have quite bad varicose veins. Am I likely to get them too?

A Why some people get them and others don't is still a mystery but some families do seem to pass on a tendency to have weak valves which can encourage the formation of varicose veins.

Q **I injured my leg in a fall recently and the doctor said I had phlebitis. Just what does that mean?**

A It is simply inflammation in the veins and is often caused by injury. It causes the blood to clot within the vein and these clots can be carried anywhere within the body.

Q **How is phlebitis treated?**

A Usually with antibiotics or simple anti-inflammation drugs and plenty of rest.

Q **The doctor has arranged for me to have an operation for an aneurysm. Is this fairly common?**

A Aneurysms are not uncommon, especially in older people.

Q **How do aneurysms develop?**

A Aneurysms are 'blow outs' of the artery wall. Arteries carry blood at high pressure round the body and their walls are fairly thick and tough in healthy people. If the artery wall loses its muscle a 'blow out' forms. The bigger the 'blow out' the greater the risk that the weak area will give way. The presence of an aneurysm means that the particular artery in which it occurs is liable to have a 'blow out' at any time.

Q **How is an aneurysm repaired?**

A It depends on where the aneurysm is located but treatment is by surgery.

Q **What does surgery for an aneurysm consist of?**

A The aneurysm can be repaired with either a vein graft, taken from another part of the body, or with one of the new man-made fibres which are incredibly strong.

Q **My mother has just been diagnosed as having gangrene. I thought that was something you only got from exposure to severe cold?**

A Anything which stops the blood supply can cause gangrene, cold is just one thing which can do this.

Q **Who is more likely to suffer from gangrene?**

A By far the largest group of sufferers from gangrene in the UK are people who develop blockage in the arteries, usually those supplying the legs. This causes chronic poor blood supply and is often associated with both atheroscerlosis and diabetes.

Q **I am quite a heavy smoker and the doctor said this may have contributed to my gangrene. Is this true?**

A Gangrene is certainly much commoner in smokers than non-smokers.

Q **What treatment is there for gangrene?**

A Once gangrene has developed the tissue is dead and the only hope is to contain the damage. Often the dead area will seal itself like a giant scab and the dead tissue will drop off. If gangrene is extensive then much tissue will have to be removed, even apparently healthy skin.

Q **Is there any chance of avoiding gangrene?**

A If severe damage to the arteries is detected in time gangrene may be avoided by medical or surgical treatment to improve the blood supply to the affected part.

Q **When I hang the washing out in the winter my fingers go all colours of the rainbow — first blue, then red and finally white! I lose all sensation in my hands and they look quite dreadful. What is causing this?**

A It could be Raynaud's Disease or Phenomenon. The condition involves uncontrollable spasm of the small blood vessels in response to cold. Whilst hands are more affected than any other part of the body, the feet, ears and face may also have the same problem to a greater or lesser degree.

Q **What can I do to lessen the discomfort in my hands when they are affected by Raynaud's Phenomenon?**

A A simple self-help measure would be to hang the washing out wearing warm sheepskin gloves. You may feel it looks odd, but it will give you some protection from the cold which is triggering the attack.

Q **What medical treatment is there for Raynaud's Phenomenon?**

A There are drugs available which help to keep the blood circulating by dilating the blood vessels, although they may have some side effects. Long-term treatment may require surgical intervention to cut the nerve supply to the blood vessels. Where possible it is far preferable to try to manage the condition without resorting to these measures.

Q **I have had Raynaud's Phenomenon for a number of years and wonder what I can do myself to try and control the problem.**

A The best remedy is to keep as active as possible, have a sensible programme of daily exercise and on no account to smoke as this can cause even more blood vessel disease. Avoid sudden changes in temperature and keep out the cold. Do not expose the hands or other affected parts during the winter and this will go a long way towards controlling the problem.

Q **I have been told that the swelling of my ankles is due to oedema. What is this?**

A Oedema is a term for fluid. It gets trapped in between the actual body cells, and is quite different from the large collections of fluid which can occur around the joints, for example, after an accident or with arthritis.

Q **When I go on a long journey my ankles always swell up. Is this unusual?**

A It is very common for fluid to get trapped around the ankles and the usual cause is sitting still for long periods, as you do on train or coach journeys.

Q **Can I do anything to help my oedema, besides just taking the tablets I have been prescribed?**

A Two simple things you can do are to put your feet up when you are sitting down and to increase the amount of exercise you do. Swimming is excellent, but anything which increases the blood flow through the legs should help to draw out the excess fluid.

Respiratory system

Q **What is catarrh?**

A Catarrh is a thick mucus discharge which usually comes from the sinuses and can be very difficult to treat.

Q **I get very bad catarrh. What can I do to cure it?**

A Initially simple inhalations of menthol, or something similar, may do the trick. If the condition persists your doctor may suggest using a nasal spray, followed by sinus investigation.

Q **Where are the sinuses?**

A The sinuses are four sets of air-filled cavities leading directly from the nose.

Q **What are the sinuses for?**

A They have two main functions. By replacing bone with air, the sinuses make the head much lighter, and therefore more easy to keep upright. Secondly, they act as resonance boxes for the voice.

Q **I think I may have sinusitis, but am not sure what causes it?**

A The problem with sinuses is that the mucus that is normally made has to be drained out through tiny openings into the nose. If the opening is blocked, when we have a cold for instance, then the mucus is trapped. This stagnant mucus very rapidly becomes infected, and then you have sinusitis.

Q **What should I look for in trying to identify sinusitis?**

A The symptoms are heaviness over the eyebrows, pain across the cheeks, and a thick yellow mucus discharge from the nose.

Q **What can I do to help myself when I have sinusitis?**

A First, stay indoors if it's winter and try to keep in an even temperature. Avoid dry air if you can because central heating can aggravate this condition. A humidifier, or just a bowl of water near a radiator, can help to put moisture back into the air. Inhalations of decongestants in a bowl of boiling water may also help.

Q **At what point should I go and see the doctor if I think I have sinusitis?**

A If there is no sign of it clearing up in a couple of days then you need to see a doctor. S/he will give you antibiotics and much stronger decongestants.

Q **I have had antibiotics for my sinusitis but it doesn't seem to be clearing up. What can I do now?**

A If your sinuses are very chronically infected then they may need washing out, or a special drainage operation, once the infection has cleared.

Q **I have been taking steroids for several months for severe asthma. I feel much better and would like to stop taking them. Should I tell my doctor or is it all right just to stop?**

A You must discuss this with your doctor first, because it is not advisable to suddenly stop taking steroids. Whatever the reason for your taking steroids, they have been preventing your own body from making these essential chemicals. If you stop suddenly then your body will not be able to cope and you may become quite ill.

Q **How should I stop taking my steroid tablets?**

A If your doctor agrees to a change in treatment s/he will advise you on how to reduce the dosage slowly — over many weeks or even months. If you subsequently get an illness or need an operation, within two years of stopping steroids, then you must immediately restart taking them, or increase the dose if you are taking a reduced amount. If you are ill then you must be sure to tell any medical attendant when you took steroids and what the dosage was. Keep a clear record of this, both on your person and at home, so the information is immediately available.

Q **What causes snoring?**

A It is caused because the throat muscles relax and, when air is breathed in or out, parts of the throat vibrate and cause the familiar noise associated with snoring.

Q Is there anything you can do to prevent snoring?

A Most sufferers sleep on their back and it helps to move them with a judicious elbow so that they are lying on their side or stomach. There are several devices available now which are worn by the snorer and emit a low electrical charge when the noise begins. This is usually sufficient to move the sleeper and stop the snoring.

Q I have to take medication for hay fever but I find it makes me very drowsy. I have to take some important exams this summer and I am worried I shall be affected. Is there anything I can do about this?

A For short-term treatment there are new antihistamines on the market which, while being very effective, do not cause drowsiness. Discuss with your doctor, or pharmacist, which would be the best for you to take.

Q I always seem to get hay fever every year. Is there anything I can do to prevent it?

A You could ask your doctor about taking a course of desensitizing injections. You have to start these early in the year to be effective during the summer period but it might prove to be worthwhile.

Q I seem to get quite a number of colds, but the doctor doesn't prescribe antibiotics. Why is this?

A A cold is an infection of the upper respiratory tract and is caused by a virus. Contrary to popular belief, antibiotics are not effective against viruses. They will only be prescribed for use against bacteria, generally if there is a secondary infection of the throat or chest.

Q I got an important new job this year where I am on the go all the time. I seem to be getting one cold after another. Is the change of job anything to do with getting colds?

A A new job can make you more vulnerable to colds because the stress that accompanies any major change does reduce your resistance to virus infections.

Q I have just moved to a new flat, which I share with two other girls, both of whom are smokers. Could the change of environment be a reason for my getting more colds than usual?

A It could be your new flatmates' habits that are causing you a problem. If you are in a smoky atmosphere, or smoke yourself, it will increase your chances of catching a cold.

Q Why do smokers get more colds than non-smokers?

A If you smoke then the whole respiratory system is constantly under attack. If there is any irritation or inflammation there already, then your body's immune system will be less able to defend itself against the cold virus. Smoking also makes cold symptoms worse by prolonging the life of a cold and encouraging an atmosphere where secondary symptoms such as bronchitis can occur.

Q Does taking medicine make a cold go away any quicker?

A Taking cold remedies will not make any difference to the length of time you have a cold, but they can alleviate some of the symptoms.

Q **My mother used to tell me to feed a cold and starve a fever. Is it just an old wives' tale?**

A Not at all, it is sound sense. During a fever you use up a lot of calories generating all that heat. If you eat a lot (though you are rarely hungry) you will fuel the fever and help it to continue.

Q **A girl in our office always comes to work when she has a cold. She says she's not contagious for the first few days, but a lot of people always seem to get colds after she's had one.**

A Not everyone does spread their germs around, but generally the first three days of a cold are when you are passing on most of the virus through contact with other people.

Q **When there is a cold going round I always seem to get it but the woman I share an office with always stays healthy. How does she do it?**

A Your friend has more resistance than you. There are a lot of reasons for this, previous infections, present good health — all these factors play a part.

Q **What is the difference between colds and 'flu?**

A A special 'Influenza' virus causes 'flu. There is almost always a high temperature, headache and joint pains, and a slight runny nose. A cold is quite different — there is rarely fever or joint pains, just a runny nose and streaming eyes and sneezing to start and stuffiness to finish.

Q What is the best treatment for 'flu?

A Stay in bed and drink plenty of fluids, at least four to six pints a day. You should keep yourself warm, but don't let the bedroom get too stuffy. You need fresh air but obviously don't want to be in a draught. If you really have no appetite at all then add some glucose to your fluid intake.

Q What's the best thing to bring my temperature down when I get 'flu?

A You can take paracetamol or soluble aspirin to help bring the temperature down and relieve the aches and pains.

Q If I have 'flu, how long should I wait before calling the doctor?

A The worst symptoms should be over in two to four days but if you still have a fever after that, then you should call in the doctor.

Q For the last few years I have had really bad bouts of 'flu that have really dragged me down. They seem to stay in my chest for ages. Is there any point in having 'flu jabs?

A Unfortunately, although the symptoms for 'flu are the same, the viruses that cause it can be quite different. The present vaccines offer protection against three of the most common strains of virus and are certainly a help, especially if you suffer from chest complaints, but they won't be effective against any new strain of virus.

Q **My mother has emphysema, which I understand is a chronic lung disease, but she looks so healthy. What is wrong with her?**

A Emphysema is a disease in which the lungs lose their elasticity. This usually results from many attacks of bronchitis or asthma in the past. The lungs remain blown up with 'dead' air containing no oxygen. This condition often leads to a classic 'barrel chest' physique which looks deceptively healthy.

Q **What can a patient with emphysema do to help themselves?**

A Although it is a progressive disease, that progress can be halted or delayed. Giving up smoking is the first thing to do, it is the most common chemical hazard to the lungs — far greater than any industrial hazard. You should avoid a dry atmosphere so if you have central heating then it is a good idea to also have humidifiers. Slightly damp air helps more rapid transfer of oxygen. Heights are also to be avoided. At the top of hills and mountains the concentration of oxygen is greatly diminished. This may be sufficient to cause even a stabilized patient severe respiratory problems.

Q **Are there any exercises that will make emphysema more bearable?**

A If you can keep the breathing muscles working as well as they possibly can, then this will certainly help the condition. Gentle exercise all over can help too, such as stretching and muscle strengthening, just as long as you do not get breathless.

Q **What causes pneumonia?**

A Pneumonia is caused by infection from bacteria, viruses or any other invading organism. If left untreated, the lungs can fill up with fluid and become waterlogged.

Q **I thought pneumonia was entirely treatable, but two people in my home town have died of it recently. Neither of them was particularly elderly, so why should this have happened?**

A With the introduction of modern antibiotics, which are very effective against bacteria, pneumonia is usually cured long before the condition becomes serious. However, viruses are not responsive to antibiotics and neither are some other types of air infection that are caused by yeasts. These can take hold in a person already debilitated by other illness. For example a cancer sufferer, or someone whose immune system is not working properly, is much less likely to be able to combat these infections of the lungs and will die from a condition which would hardly cause a fit person a day off work. People who are already sick are much more susceptible to pneumonia. The healthy majority do not have to worry about it at all.

Q **What are the benefits of breathing through the nose?**

A The nose has a very delicate lining which in normal circumstances makes a small amount of fine mucus which lies suspended in the nose by a bed of fine hairs. This system is geared to filtering the air we breathe and it is very efficient at its job. Particles of dust and some bacteria and other bugs are trapped in this mucus and destroyed, so preventing them from getting down into our lungs.

Q Ever since I can remember I have breathed through my mouth. My husband says this is unhealthy, but does it really make any difference?

A The mouth has no filtering system, like the nose, so dust particles and germs can get into the lungs without hindrance. Breathing through your mouth is more likely to lead you to suffer from coughs and colds than the normal 'nose breathers'.

Q I have been an asthmatic from childhood and was never able to play any sports at school. When I do any form of exercise I have great difficulty breathing, although I am all right at other times. I know how important it is to try and keep fit, but is there any sport at all that I could get involved in?

A You have a type of exercise-induced asthma and, although sufferers get very breathless in most exercise activities, it does seem that swimming does not bring on the same symptoms. It has perhaps to do with the dampness of the air around all that water. In the UK, the Asthma Swim Movement has been created to help people like you and they have groups throughout the country who meet regularly.

Q My husband gave up smoking three years ago and is always on at me to do the same. I can understand why he gave up because men are more prone to heart attacks, but surely it's not dangerous for me?

A Although heart disease appears to be less common in young women than in men of the same age, once you are through the menopause then heart attacks are every bit as common in women as in men — particularly in smokers. Also, in older women, apart from heart disease, lung cancer deaths are increasing dramatically.

Q **My mother has suffered badly from bronchitis for a number of years and is on medicines constantly. She sleeps with her window open all through the winter and I am sure this is not good for her. Am I right?**

A Cold, damp places should be avoided at all costs, and the tradition of sleeping with the window open will not help her condition at all.

Q **In winter I usually get at least one attack of bronchitis. I worry about staying off work, do I really need to be at home?**

A Yes, you really should stay away from work and apart from other people. Although you may not feel too bad, the problem is that you could spread the germs to others.

Q **What treatment will I be given for bronchitis?**

A You may be given either tablets or sprays (called bronchodilators) which work to counteract the narrowing or spasm of the bronchial tubes caused by the infection. Cough suppressants are also very useful.

Q **Can I do anything myself to make the bronchitis easier?**

A If it is a mild case you should keep your room warm, but not stuffy. A bowl of water will often stop the air from drying out and inhalations can soothe and control the tiresome and painful cough.

Q **I know I really should give up smoking but I don't seem to have any will-power. Can any of the alternative therapies help?**

A The most important thing in getting any technique to work is for you to really want to give up. If you do, then there are many ways to go about it. Some tried and tested methods include hypnosis, acupuncture, aversion therapy, chewing gum and many more. Just pick one and stick to it!

Blood

Blood is the vital substance that flows through the body, carrying oxygen and nutrients and removing waste materials from the tissues. It makes up around a fourteenth of our body weight. The average adult carries five litres, or eight pints, of blood in their system.

Q **What is high blood cholesterol?**

A Cholesterol is one of the fatty substances present in the blood and all body tissues. If your blood cholesterol is high it simply means that you have more than is normal and there may then be a gradual build-up of fatty deposits in the body. This can lead to a greater risk of developing coronary heart disease.

Q **What does anaemia mean?**

A It is a blanket term that can cover many conditions. It indicates that either the number or quality (or both) of the red blood cells is diminished. We need a good supply of these cells and they must be well filled with an iron-containing compound called haemoglobin. It is this compound which enables oxygen to be carried around in the blood stream and reach every cell in our bodies, allowing it to 'breathe' and function properly.

Q **What causes pernicious anaemia?**

A It is due to a deficiency of vitamin B12.

Q **How do we become deficient in vitamin B12?**

A Normally we are able to make enough of this vitamin from our food, but sometimes the chemical reactions in the stomach, which are necessary to create it, fail. Vitamin B12 is poorly absorbed from tablets, so if we fail to make our own it must be injected directly into the bloodstream. Usually a dose once a month is all that is necessary.

Q **My parents originally came from Cyprus and I have just learned that I have a tendency for a type of anaemia called thalassaemia. Is there anything I can do about this?**

A No, there is nothing you can do. This tendency, or trait, is inherited and you cannot alter it. It will almost certainly give you no problems. Unless of course you happen to pick a partner who has exactly the same trait as you. Then you will have a one in four chance of having a child affected by the full-blown disease of thalassaemia major.

Q We are going to visit our daughter in West Africa soon and I am quite concerned about the AIDS problem. I know that you can get it from blood transfusions and dirty needles, so what happens if we are taken ill out there?

A It is not just AIDS that you can catch if you have blood transfusions and injections, there are other diseases like hepatitis that can occur if the equipment or blood has not been properly treated. If you are concerned, you can get a sterile equipment pack which includes sterile syringes, needles, swabs and plasters to take away with you. Your doctor will be able to advise you.

Q How often should I have tetanus injections? I am a keen gardener and am always getting cuts and scratches from weeding and pruning.

A The initial course of anti-tetanus shots is of three separate injections, with six weeks between the first two and six months between the second two. Ideally you should have a tetanus booster not less than one year after you have completed your full initial course of immunisations. The most risky situations for contracting tetanus are where the soil has been contaminated with animal faeces. This usually applies to most gardens where manure is regularly used as a fertilizer. It is dangerous because the tetanus spores can survive for many years in such soil.

Q My husband is a haemophiliac. He has occasional blood product injections to maintain his good health but otherwise he lives a normal life. We would eventually like to have a family, but what are the chances of his haemophilia being passed on?

A Your children will not have haemophilia, but your grandchildren may.

Q How is haemophilia carried?

A Haemophilia is an inherited disease, but it is very special in that the affected gene is carred on the X chromosome — the female one. Every normal man has an X chromosome — in your husband's case a haemophiliac one — and a Y chromosome. When you have children, your chromosomes and those of your husband mix. Any girls must have your husband's tainted X chromosome and a normal X from you — they will not be affected because the normal X overrides the tainted one. Any boys will have a normal Y chromosome from your husband and a normal X from you — so they will not have haemophilia either. Unless by a very rare fluke his wife also carries a tainted X chromosome, the children of a haemophiliac man never have the disease — however his grandchildren may have. If his daughter carries one of the tainted X chromosomes she may pass it to her son — and he *would* be a haemophiliac.

Q Is it true that being a blood donor will help you to live a longer life?

A Blood donors are certainly necessary in modern day medicine and there is no indication that being a blood donor does any harm to a normal, healthy person. There is no concrete evidence that it helps you live longer either, but by diluting your blood from time to time and keeping your bone marrow active it may help to keep you well. In the past, blood letting was considered very good treatment, and is still used in some areas today.

Q **Whenever I have a cold I get a nosebleed and I seem to lose a lot of blood. Is this usual?**

A During a cold the delicate lining of the nose gets damaged by the constant blowing and wiping, and a scab forms over the damaged area. If the scab is dislodged by further vigorous blowing then the base of the scab will bleed. The amount of blood can seem quite out of proportion because a great number of tiny blood vessels become dilated during an acute cold.

Q **What is the best way to treat a nosebleed?**

A First sit *forward* and let the blood drip into a bowl or onto tissues. Then grip the whole of the soft cartilage end of your nose between your thumb and finger and *pinch firmly*, breathing all the time through your mouth. Sit calmly for a few minutes and gradually release the pressure to see what happens. If the blood is still flowing freely then reapply pressure. Normally the blood will clot and a scab will form over the damaged area within a minute or two.

Q **Over the past few months I have had quite a few nosebleeds and was wondering whether to see the doctor?**

A It is important to have frequent nosebleeds checked out by your doctor. Occasionally very high blood pressure will cause nose bleeds and so can certain forms of anaemia. Locally, polyps in the nose or other growths can cause the same symptoms so it is important to get the problem properly investigated.

Digestive system

Problems with the digestive system are common to all of us at some time or other. If we are what we eat, then we seem to exist on a diet of acidity and heartburn with side dishes of constipation and wind thrown in for good measure. Sensible eating habits can do so much to make our digestive system healthy and comfortable and yet we often choose to ignore the most basic signals our body can send us to let us know when something is wrong.

The stomach and digestion

Q **After I have eaten my stomach often blows up and feels as hard as a rock. What can I do about it?**

A Basically you need to stop taking in so much air when you eat. Rapid eating is the usual cause of this problem so try slowing down and really taking your time over your food.

Q **I have a persistent pain behind my breast bone which comes on at any time. All the tests have proved normal so what should I do now?**

A This kind of intermittent problem can be very tedious, especially when you can't seem to find anything specific that is wrong. One other possibility may be an irritation at the lower end of your oesophagus, down which food travels into your stomach. This irritation can be caused by taking certain medicines or tablets like aspirin. Discuss it with your doctor and then stop taking any tablets for a week or so and see if it makes any difference.

Q Because I have been suffering from stomach pains, my doctor has told me that I need to go to the hospital for a barium meal. Why can't they just X-ray my stomach?

A The stomach and intestines do not show up on X-ray examinations in the normal course of events, unlike hard things like bones and teeth. The only way to outline your stomach is to put something inside you which will block the X-rays, and barium salts do exactly that.

Q What happens when I am given a barium meal?

A The barium salts are made up into a milky-flavoured suspension for you to drink. You are then taken to a darkened room where the radiologist can examine your stomach and take X-rays which will be studied later.

Q Is having a barium meal painful?

A It is not painful, but it can be a bit tedious if your stomach is not feeling too good.

Q Every time I eat I get a pain in my stomach. I am worried that I might have an ulcer.

A Pain in the upper part of the stomach, usually in the middle just under the rib cage, can be associated with ulcers. If it persists over a month or so then talk to your doctor about it.

Q There seem to be several kinds of ulcer. What is the difference between them?

A There are two quite separate types of peptic ulcer. Those found in the stomach are called gastric ulcers and the other group are the duodenal ulcers.

Q **Where exactly is the duodenum?**

A The duodenum is the piece of gut that joins the stomach to the rest of the lower intestine.

Q **I have got a stomach ulcer and am anxious to do as much as I can to minimize the pain and discomfort.**

A The first thing to look at is your diet. Cut out alcohol and smoking altogether and go on a regime of wholemeal bread, milk, fish, eggs and water.

Q **Surely it will help my ulcer if I just eat much less?**

A You must not allow yourself to get hungry, because the pain of an ulcer can be made worse by the acid that the stomach produces in those circumstances.

Q **What things should I look out for with an ulcer?**

A Take a bland drink such as milk to relieve it, and don't in any circumstances eat highly spiced foods or acids such as vinegar.

Q **I have only got a very small ulcer but my doctor has put me on medicines and a diet that seems to go on for ever. Do I really need to bother with it?**

A If you follow your doctor's instructions to the letter, for at least six weeks, the chances are that your ulcer will heal completely and give you no further trouble. If you do not take the symptoms seriously then the ulcer may get too big and take a long time to heal, become chronic or eventually need an operation to remove it.

Q **Why are ulcers so painful?**

A An ulcer is a breach in the lining of the stomach. The digestive juices that normally work on breaking down our food are then able to get through that breach and start acting on the tissues underneath the ulcer. This is very painful.

Q **My mother has to go into hospital for a partial gastrectomy. Please could you explain what is involved?**

A This is an operation to remove a stomach ulcer that has not been controlled through diet and medication. In a gastrectomy, approximately seven-eighths of the stomach may be taken away.

Q **I have been told that as well as a partial gastrectomy the surgeon is going to do a vagotomy. Just what is this?**

A It's an additional procedure where the nerves to the stomach are also cut to reduce the production of acid.

Q **If they're going to take away seven-eighths of my stomach, why don't they just take all of it and be done with it?**

A It is very important that some of the stomach is left behind as, without the stomach's secretions, certain vitamins cannot be produced. If this occurs, then pernicious anaemia may follow. You also need a small sac to contain your food before it passes into the gut.

Q **What exactly is the appendix?**

A The appendix is a small blind sac about two inches long attached to the lower part of the gut. It is always found in the lower right side of your abdomen.

Q **What are the symptoms of appendicitis?**

A In a very acute case the signs are fairly dramatic. If someone who is normally perfectly healthy starts to vomit and complains of pains in their stomach, accompanied by a low-grade fever, then you should get medical help.

Q **I'm not sure where the pain is when you have appendicitis?**

A The pain can start on the left of the abdomen, or centrally over the navel and need not be constant, sometimes it can disappear for up to an hour or so. In a really acute case the pain may be so severe that it makes the sufferer sweat and writhe around the bed, and can be accompanied by very bad breath.

Q **If I'm not sure whether or not it's appendicitis, should I call the doctor?**

A Severe or recurrent abdominal pain should always be checked. Don't just grin and bear it.

Q **My sister had an operation for a perforated appendix but I'm not sure exactly what this meant.**

A If an acutely inflamed appendix is not removed it may perforate. Then infected bowel contents are tipped into the abdomen. This gives rise to peritonitis. A large appendix abscess can form round this and take many weeks to get better. If you have an operation when an abscess is already formed it can be very troublesome indeed to heal.

Q **How long will I have to stay in hospital if I have my appendix removed?**

A Usually the day after the operation you should be out of bed and able to walk to the toilet with some help. By the fourth day after the operation you may be allowed home.

Q **When I had my appendix out last year I thought that would be the end of it, but I still get pain on that side. What could be causing it?**

A Sometimes the lymph glands around the gut get inflamed and can cause pain. The condition is called mesenteric adenitis. It is not serious but it can recur.

Q **What is peritonitis?**

A It's an inflammation of the peritoneum. This is the membrane lining which covers all the abdominal organs.

Q **Sometimes if I have had a lot to drink, whether it's wine or spirits, I vomit and it seems to be brownish in colour. Is this all right?**

A It sounds as if you are vomiting a small amount of blood and this is coming from the surface of your stomach. Alcohol can cause stomach ulcers, and this is a condition that needs to be treated. You should certainly stop drinking until you have consulted a doctor about it.

Q **What does anorexia nervosa mean?**

A Loss of appetite, due to nervous causes.

Q **My teenage daughter is very thin. Although she seems to eat quite normally, she has lost over a stone in weight. Is this anorexia?**

A If she is eating normally then it is not anorexia. However, if she is losing weight at the rate you say, then she may be making herself vomit after eating so that she doesn't keep in her food. This condition is called bulimia.

Q **I have recently taken up swimming and like to go every Sunday after lunch. My mother says you should never swim after you've eaten. Why not?**

A When you eat, the blood supply around your stomach and gut increases enormously to help digestion. If you then put lots of demands on your muscles by vigorous exercise of any sort you can get severe cramp. Cramp on dry land may be painful, but it's not dangerous; cramp in deep water with no help at hand can be fatal.

The bowels and evacuation

Q **I suffer terribly with wind and it really can be very embarrassing if I am in company. What causes it?**

A There are only two ways that wind gets into the intestine. The first is that it is swallowed during eating. Many people take in quite large amounts of air when they are eating — gulping down a cup of tea, for instance. The other way that gas gets into the stomach is by the action of bacteria on the food you eat.

Q **What can I do about an attack of wind?**

A One of the best remedies is to eat charcoal biscuits. They work by absorbing the gas and you can easily buy them at any pharmacy.

Q **I have heard that exercise can help reduce attacks of wind. Is this true?**

A Yes, exercise will tone up your stomach muscles and prevent your intestine being able to swell up so much that it holds large pockets of wind.

Q **I know it is healthy to have a 'regular' bowel movement. But how often is regular?**

A It varies enormously from one person to another. Daily would be ideal, or at least every other day, but the important thing is to have a spontaneous and unaided bowel movement.

Q **I never had any constipation until I left home and started fending for myself at college. I have a healthy diet, so what has gone wrong?**

A Leaving home can be very stressful and that might just have upset your natural rhythm. Also, time is a very important factor. If you are always rushing then you might be ignoring your body's messages about when it wants to have a bowel movement. If you keep ignoring it, then it eventually stops sending the messages.

Q **Is there anything I can do to help my bowels move every day?**

A It will help if you can establish a regular routine. Many people find first thing in the morning suits them and a glass of hot water taken first thing before breakfast seems to stimulate quite a few people into having a bowel movement.

Q **How are my bowels affected if I eat a lot of convenience foods, cakes and biscuits?**

A If you eat mostly highly refined foods, with a low-bulk content, then the amount of material to be evacuated from the bowel is greatly reduced. Because the material spends more time in the bowel much of the fluid content is absorbed and so the stool becomes hard and much smaller. This small stool fails to stimulate the bowels, either to move it along or give it the urge for evacuation and so you are constipated.

Q **The only time I seem to suffer from constipation is just before my period. Why is this?**

A In the week before your period the level of progesterone is very high and this tends to decrease the mobility of the bowel.

Q **I became a vegetarian last year and my bowel movements have changed completely. The motion is much softer and more frequent. Is this entirely due to my diet?**

A If you have a diet high in vegetables and low in animal fats then your motion will have plenty of bulk and will be easy to pass. You may also have up to two or three bowel actions a day on this kind of diet.

Q **My mother has taken a laxative every day for years. She says that without them she doesn't have a daily bowel movement, but surely it must be bad for her to take them so regularly?**

A In an ideal world nobody would need to take laxatives because their diet would ensure that their bowels moved naturally. You could suggest your mother cuts down her intake of laxatives to taking them only on alternate days, or even once a week. She will probably be resistant to this, but do persevere.

Q **I have taken laxatives for a long time but have finally stopped. How can I get my bowel to move again naturally?**

A Try to increase the amount of high-bulk foods in your diet, such as vegetables and fruit. This way you will retrain your bowel to move by itself.

Q **I know laxatives aren't a good thing to take all the time, but surely there is no harm in taking them occasionally?**

A It depends on how you define occasionally. It is preferable not to use one more than half a dozen times a year. Regular use of laxatives never solves a problem, it just creates one.

Q I have never taken laxatives. If I am constipated I just have a good curry and a bottle of wine and that seems to do the trick!

A Curry and alcohol are both stimulants and do stir the bowels into action. Just be sure you don't overdo it.

Q I am not sure what sort of laxative I need. Where can I get advice?

A Different sorts of laxatives do have different actions, and which one you choose will depend on what your particular problem is. Your pharmacist will be able to give you detailed advice, but there are three main types; bulk, stimulant, and softening.

Q I had been using a laxative only occasionally, but when I became pregnant the doctor told me to stop using it. Why was this?

A It was probably a stimulant laxative that you were using. These work by irritating the bowel wall and increasing bowel mobility. They act quickly, but if your bowel material is hard and dry then there can be the risk of a tear to the anal skin when the motion is expelled. The chemicals contained in these laxatives make them unsuitable for nursing mothers because they can be passed on into the breast milk.

Q When I was little my grandmother used to give me liquid paraffin every day 'to keep me regular'. Did it really have any effect or was it just an old wives' tale?

A Yes it does have an effect. Liquid paraffin softens the motion and makes it easier to pass. It can be very helpful for those whose stools are very hard.

Q My doctor told me just to add bran to my breakfast cereal, to help with my constipation. I took it for a couple of days, but didn't notice any difference.

A Bran is one of the commonest bulk laxatives and acts by increasing the volume of material in the bowel, stimulating it in a gentle way. The stool is larger and softer but may not be passed for two or three days. You need to persevere for a bit longer to see results.

Q My doctor told me that I have an anal fissure. What is this?

A Simply, a fissure is a tear in the anal skin which opens up again each and every time there is a bowel movement. Naturally, as this is so very painful, patients try to avoid visits to the lavatory and thus end up even more constipated.

Q Are some people more likely to get anal fissures than others?

A It is a condition that often occurs in patients with haemorrhoids.

Q What treatment will I be given for an anal fissure?

A The treatment will depend on how severe the fissure is, and whether or not you also have haemorrhoids. The first step is normally an injection of a local anaesthetic to take the pain away. Then medicines to make the bowel movements soft, so that it is easily passed without straining. If these steps are not successful then an operation is required.

Q **What exactly are piles and how do they develop?**

A Quite simply a pile, or haemorrhoid, is a varicose vein of the back passage. A bout of constipation can start them off and straining to pass a motion will make them worse.

Q **What treatment should I have for haemorrhoids?**

A Haemorrhoids are not permanent in most people and with special attention to bowel habits they will get better. If there is a fissure or crack accompanying the condition then there will also be pain and it is important to get this treated properly. It is important to keep the anus clean and there are special medicated wipes you can get for this purpose. The best treatment though is to ensure that you are regularly passing soft motions, easily and without strain. To do this you should ensure that you eat plenty of high-bulk food such as fruit and vegetables and have at least two to three glasses of water every day.

Q **My haemorrhoids are quite painful but my doctor said I shouldn't take any codeine for them. Why was this?**

A It is essential that you do not take painkillers that decrease bowel action, such as codeine, because you will be increasing the constipation and making the haemorrhoids even worse.

Q **I have noticed some slight bleeding recently when I have a bowel movement. Should I see the doctor about it?**

A Bleeding from the back passage is always a cause for concern and, however slight, should always be reported to your doctor.

Q **My bowel motions have suddenly become very dark and sometimes there is a trace of blood. What is causing this?**

A If you are taking oral iron tablets then this can cause your motions to appear almost black. *But*, apart from this single condition, if you notice blood — or your bowel movements are very dark — then you should consult a doctor at once to discuss the problem.

Q **I have just started a new job that involves quite a bit of foreign travel. What can I take that will help with 'traveller's tummy'?**

A Most travellers' diarrhoea is caused by a common bacteria — E coli. Simple antibiotics are effective against this organism but in most cases the diarrhoea will get better without any treatment. You could carry one of the anti-diarrhoea medicines that are available from a pharmacist. That will control the immediate problem.

Q **What can I do to help myself when I have diarrhoea?**

A If you have an attack make sure that you drink plenty of fluids — but not alcohol. You must be scrupulous about washing your hands every time you use the lavatory, prepare food, handle plates or cutlery. Do not use a teatowel or dishcloth but wash everything under running water and leave to dry in the air.

Q **Why shouldn't you drink alcohol if you've had diarrhoea?**

A Alcohol pulls water out of the body and can never be used to replace fluid lost during a diarrhoea attack.

Q **If I have diarrhoea, how long should I wait before consulting a doctor?**

A Any diarrhoea that has not shown any signs of improving after 48 hours should be referred to a doctor.

Q **If I get an attack of diarrhoea I seem to feel very weak afterwards. What causes this?**

A If there has been excessive diarrhoea over several days then you have lost a great deal of your body's necessary fluids, salt and potassium and this can make you feel weak.

Q **Is there anything I can do to counteract this loss?**

A A simple treatment to replace the fluids is to take a litre of pure, cooled, previously boiled water and add to it one teaspoonful of salt, eight teaspoonsfuls of sugar and, if you have them, add three quarters of a level teaspoonful of sodium bicarbonate and a third of a level teaspoonful of potassium chloride. This should be drunk as often as possible.

Q **I have suffered for years from an embarrassing itch around my bottom. I try not to scratch it, but it drives me crazy. Is it very common?**

A At some time or another most adults suffer from this problem and it is a self-perpetuating condition. If you itch, you scratch, the skin is then damaged and other infections can occur — leading to more itching.

Q **What can I do to stop this itching?**

A Keep the skin around the bottom scrupulously clean by washing night and morning and after every bowel action. Soap stings, so try to keep it to a minimum and wash it off thoroughly, but do not use a flannel.

Q **The toilet paper I use seems to make my skin itch worse. What can I do about it?**

A Instead of toilet paper use skin wipes (such as those for babies), but make sure they do not contain surgical spirit.

Q **My doctor said I should dry myself with a hairdryer after I've been to the lavatory. Surely she was joking?**

A No, it was a sensible suggestion. Bacteria and other germs like warm moist places to grow in so it's necessary to make sure you dry the skin thoroughly after wiping and washing. If you have a hairdryer in your bathroom then that is an excellent way to get the skin really dry.

Q **Will different kinds of clothing make the itching worse?**

A It's best if you avoid tight jeans or any type of girdle, because they can press the buttocks together and aid infection. If you wear loose clothes and cotton pants then that should help.

Q **I've been using talcum powder to keep my skin dry, because I sweat such a lot. Is any type of powder all right to use?**

A Don't use ordinary talcum or baby powder in the affected area. Your pharmacist will be able to recommend a special drying powder which is more suitable. If you sweat a lot then put some of the powder onto a thin pad of cotton wool, or panty liner, and leave in place over your anal skin between washes.

Q **Will it help with my itching if I put some cream around my anus?**

A You should avoid most ointments and creams, unless your doctor has prescribed them, because they will keep the skin soggy and moist and may cause some allergic reactions. If the skin is broken then you may need a special antiseptic lotion and your doctor will prescribe one.

Q **Does being constipated make any difference to my itching?**

A It will help if you can try to make sure your bowel motions are regular and that you avoid any constipation. If there is anything which you know can cause you to have diarrhoea, then avoid that too.

Q **The itch on my skin is driving me mad. It seems to be worse at night. What can I do?**

A At all costs you must avoid scratching or it will get worse. If you wear cotton gloves in bed, they will prevent you scratching yourself in your sleep.

Q **I think I may have worms but am too embarrassed to go to the doctor. What can I do?**

A Your doctor will not think anything about it at all. After all, worms are often caught through no fault of your own. If you really can't face your doctor, then your pharmacist can direct you to a suitable product which can be bought over the counter.

Q **What can I do to avoid getting worms?**

A Always wash your hands immediately before and after handling food. This is the best way of protecting against worm infestation.

Q **What is colitis?**

A True colitis is an inflammation of the bowel.

Q **I have been told I have ulcerative colitis. What exactly is this?**

A It is a condition in which the colon is chronically inflamed and ulcerated. In it's very acute phase there may even be perforations of the bowel wall and large abscesses can form.

Q **My sister has ulcerative colitis. What sort of treatment will she be given?**

A Treatment is usually by steroid tablets and antibiotics, especially in the acute stages. In some cases surgery may be necessary to remove the affected part of the colon.

Q **Is ulcerative colitis very common?**

A Ulcerative colitis affects about one in every 1500 people.

Q **I know Crohn's disease affects the bowel, but how do you recognize it?**

A Crohn's disease shows itself as an acute inflammation of the bowel and any part of the large or small bowel can be affected.

Q **Although I am only 22 I have had Crohn's disease for six years. I have had one operation but nobody seems able to tell me exactly what causes it.**

A The bowel wall responds just as though it was suffering from an acute infection, but — and here lies the problem — there has been no infection or allergy producing agent which has yet been properly identified. Unfortunately it is not yet possible to say what causes this condition.

Q **I'm not sure what colostomy and ileostomy mean?**

A Stoma means hole. Both a colostomy and an ileostomy are artificial holes made in different parts of the gut. An ileostomy is a hole in the middle gut (or ileum), and a colostomy is a hole in the lower gut (or colon).

Q What is the difference between a colostomy and an ileostomy operation?

A Normally waste products are passed down the gut and expelled from the body at the anus. The gut is an enormously long tube, more than 30 feet in length, and if any of it becomes diseased, quite large chunks can be removed and the ends joined together without the patient having any special problems. However, if there is a disease of the lower bowel, rectum or anus, this joining up procedure is just not possible and an artificial opening for the gut has to be made on the front of the abdomen. If the lower gut (or colon) opens on to the surface it is called a colostomy, if it is the middle gut (or ileum) it is an ileostomy.

Q Why is my mother so embarrassed about having a colostomy? I cannot get her to talk to me about it at all.

A Coping with a colostomy can be a very traumatic experience. Instead of visits to the lavatory being discreet and out of sight, the motion will be passed right in front where it is easy to see. This can be difficult to adjust to, so give your mother time to feel more comfortable about the idea. Your doctor may know whether there is a local counselling service for people who have had colostomies or ileostomies, so that she can talk to other people who have had the operation.

Q I am concerned about how I'll manage after my colostomy. I am worried about dealing with my bowel contents.

A Specialist nurses are trained to teach patients how to use the collecting bags efficiently and they will happily answer any questions and put your mind at rest. Nowadays it is a very clean and tidy procedure and you really do not need to be worried.

Q **I have had a colostomy for many years now since I had my lower bowel removed because of cancer. I do find wearing a colostomy bag very tedious, are there any new ways of managing this condition?**

A There is a small disposable mushroom-shaped plug which can be used for *stable* colostomies for up to twelve hours at a time. It is available on prescription so do ask your doctor about it.

Q **I have been told I have diverticulitis. What exactly is it?**

A Diverticulum simply means 'blind sac' and what happens is that a number of these sacs develop along the length of the bowel tube. They are formed around the colon where there are areas of weakness in the muscles and sacs of greater or lesser size are allowed to form. These sacs have narrow openings into the main bowel and can easily get clogged up with debris from the gut. Diverticulosis is the name given to the condition when no infection is present.

Q **Is diverticulitis common?**

A Yes, it's very common as we get older and women are more likely to be affected than men.

Q **What causes diverticulitis?**

A Diverticulitis is the name given when the diverticulum, or sac, becomes infected. 'Itis' on the end of a word always means inflammation and probable infection. Just one, or all, of the sacs may be infected. The commonest cause for these sacs to form is constipation.

Q **Is it true that a poor diet can lead to diverticulitis?**

A It is thought that when the bowel contents are stagnated, possibly because they contain little bulk in the form of fibre, this helps the formation of diverticula.

Q **What are the symptoms of diverticulitis?**

A Because each sac acts like a miniature appendix, the infection can lead to a great deal of pain. An abscess can form around the infection and, in severe cases, the diverticulum can burst and peritonitis can result.

Q **What treatment is available for diverticulitis?**

A Generally, antibiotics are prescribed and whilst the attack lasts it is best to rest the bowel as much as possible by only taking in fluids. You should have as many bland and glucose-containing drinks as you can manage.

Q **Will the diverticulitis go away on it's own, or am I stuck with it?**

A It is a permanent condition because it is based on a change in the actual appearance of the colon.

Q **What can I do to help my diverticulitis?**

A Apart from removing the whole colon, which is a major operation, you cannot get rid of the sacs once they have formed. What you can do is keep the diverticula healthy by having a good diet that includes plenty of fibre, exercising regularly and keeping your weight at its ideal level.

Q **Why do I need to keep my weight down because I have diverticulitis?**

A It is important to avoid becoming overweight because obesity seems to play a part in the development of diverticula, perhaps because fatty deposits in and around the gut weaken the muscles.

Organs and glands

The largest organ in the body is the liver. It plays an important part in fat and protein metabolism and converts sugar into glycogen, which it then stores. The bladder and kidneys can cause problems for many women, because the urethra — the connecting tube between the bladder and the outside world — is shorter than in men and gives less protection against bacteria entering. This can give rise to infections such as cystitis.

Bladder and kidneys

Q **I have a very embarrassing problem which I find difficult to discuss with my doctor. Every time I run for a bus, or cough or sneeze, I leak a small amount of urine. It is not much, but enough to wet my pants. Why does this happen?**

A It is called stress incontinence. It is not related to emotional stress, but the sudden increase of pressure that stresses the muscles which control the bladder. If they are weak then there is a possibility that urine will escape.

Q **How rare is it for women to suffer from stress incontinence?**

A It is a very common condition and over 50 per cent of women will experience this problem at some time in their adult life.

Q **Can certain foods or drinks make incontinence worse?**

A If you have an unstable bladder then it may be aggravated by caffeine (as found in tea, coffee and cola) and alcohol. For some people cold weather, or the sound of running water, is sufficient to cause them problems.

Q **Is there anything I can do about stress incontinence without seeing my doctor?**

A There are self-help measures that will improve the muscles around your bladder, but if there is no improvement at all after you have tried them for a couple of weeks you should go to your doctor for a full check-up. First, make a regular practice of pulling up the muscles of your pelvic floor and holding them tight. Then when you go to the lavatory try to stop the flow of urine by using your muscles to hold it back, count to four and then release. Practice releasing and holding back so that you have control over the flow and this will greatly strengthen the muscles around your urethra.

When you have the sensation of being able to control those muscles, then practice tightening and releasing them regularly throughout the day. Ideally four times an hour, every hour, whether you're watching television or washing the dishes. If you keep this routine up for at least three months then you should see very positive results.

Q **Although I am now 35 I still wet myself occasionally at night. I find it very embarrassing and wonder if there is any point in seeing my doctor, as I have had this habit since I was a child.**

A As this problem is so persistent you really should seek help from your doctor. The surgery may have a practice nurse whom you might prefer to talk to first. Whatever the cause, physical or psychological, your doctor will be able to suggest some treatment for you. Often tablets which will stop you sleeping too deeply are all that is necessary.

Q **What causes cystitis?**

A Cystitis is a whole range of problems that relate to the urinary bladder. The commonest type of cystitis is caused by bacteria. These like warm, moist places and billions upon billions of them live in the intestines of each and every one of us in the normal course of events. By the very nature of a woman's anatomy quite a few of these bacteria get onto the surface of the skin around the opening of the vagina and urethra. Normally these bacteria are kept in check by normal healthy skin, but if there is a tiny cut or scratch or any other damage to the skin then infections can easily gain entry to the bladder.

Q **I keep getting attacks of cystitis, is there anything I can do to prevent them?**

A Yes, there are a few behavioural changes that can make a lot of difference to cystitis sufferers. You need to keep the kidneys working well and flush out the urethra, so every day you should drink several glasses of plain water. Proper toilet hygiene is vital too, always wipe from front to back — never wipe the bladder area after wiping the anus. Intercourse can also trigger off an attack of cystitis and it can be helpful to empty your bladder beforehand — this makes sure that the bladder and urethra are not bruised — and afterwards too — this will flush out any bacteria that have got into the urethra.

Q **Is there anything the doctor can prescribe to help with cystitis?**

A It will depend on what particular germ is causing the attack, but there are several things that can help. You may be given a mild alkali, like potassium citrate (Mist Pot. Cit.), to reduce the pain and burning of passing water. If the attack is more severe then sulphonamides or other antibiotics may be given to kill off the bacteria.

Q **Are there things I can do to help myself during an attack of cystitis?**

A During an attack drink water with a teaspoon of sodium bicarbonate dissolved in it, every hour until the pain has gone. A predominantly liquid diet for a day or two may be helpful. You should avoid drinks like tea, coffee and cola as they contain caffeine and this could aggravate the condition. Chlorinated water and citrus fruit juices are also irritants to cystitis so if possible stick to filtered or spring water and herb teas.

Q **I have been taking diuretics for quite a few years now to control my weight. Is there any harm in it?**

A Water retention is very rarely the true explanation of being overweight. Only in severe heart or kidney disease is enough water retained to make more than a few pounds worth of difference. Diuretics are a group of drugs which work by pulling excess water out of the body and their long-term use can blunt the ability of the kidneys to respond to normal circumstances. Do discuss this with your doctor and ask for help to come off these tablets.

Q **My sister needs to have a kidney transplant and I would like to offer myself as donor. How would giving up one of my kidneys affect me?**

A We all have two kidneys, but in fact really only need about half of one to manage most of our everyday needs. If you are in normal health then it is perfectly possible for you to donate one of your kidneys without your own needs being affected. However, it is not a decision to be taken lightly and you should talk it over carefully with both your sister and her medical advisers. It may even be that you are not a suitable match for your sister — she would then reject your kidney and no one would benefit.

Liver and spleen

Q **I am not sure exactly how my liver processes food in the body. Can you explain?**

A The liver is really a complicated chemical factory. It breaks down partially digested food into the simplest forms of protein, fat and carbohydrate and then builds them up into different combinations which the human body needs. It also breaks down waste chemicals and any medicines or drugs we take (including alcohol) so they can be cleared out of the body.

Q **Why do people with jaundice go yellow?**

A The liver processes a chemical called bilirubin, made in the normal break down of red blood cells. It is a yellowish pigment that normally exists in the body but if too much of it is in the blood the excess shows up in our skin and eyes, which are stained yellow. Too much bilirubin is made if blood is broken down excessively, as in malaria, or if excretion through the bile ducts is blocked — for instance by a gall stone.

Q **What is hepatitis?**

A This is a very common condition and is an inflammation of the liver. It can be caused by a variety of factors but virus infection is one of the most common.

Q **What is the difference between Hepatitis A and Hepatitis B?**

A Hepatitis A and Hepatitis B are both viruses. Hepatitis A usually affects young people and children on an individual basis. There are occasional epidemics of Hepatitis A and recovery is usually complete. Hepatitis B, on the other hand, develops after direct contact with infected blood or other body secretions such as saliva or faeces. Hepatitis B is normally cleared from 90 per cent of people who suffer from it, although it may take a long time to go completely. But 10 per cent of sufferers continue to harbour the virus. They are carriers and can give hepatitis to others.

Q **I have been offered immunization against Hepatitis B by my employer. Is it worth having?**

A If you are in a high risk job, such as hospital nursing, or the accident services, then you would be well advised to get this protection. Hepatitis B can permanently damage the liver and is responsible for many thousands of deaths world-wide each year.

Q **I keep coming out in boils. I have never had them before and now, at 45, it seems embarrassing to go to the doctor about it. Will they just keep going away of their own accord?**

A Boils which start for the first time in middle or later life can be associated with early diabetes. The excess sugar in the body tissues seems to support the growth of the bacteria which causes boils. Finding out if you have diabetes is done by a simple urine test and it would be sensible to talk to your doctor so that this possibility can be checked out.

Q **What are the symptoms of diabetes?**

A Common symptoms are a much increased thirst and, associated with that, passing a great deal of urine. Young diabetics lose weight and often the first sign is a coma. In 'maturity onset' diabetes there is often a yeast infection of the skin, causing anal and vulval irritation. Other skin infections such as boils and styes are also common in diabetics.

Q **My doctor wants me to be tested for diabetes and I would like to know what is involved.**

A It is a simple test to check the urine to find out if there is any sugar in it. A stick impregnated with a special chemical is dipped into a small amount of urine and a colour change will show if there is sugar present. If this finding is positive, then a blood test will follow to establish what kind of diabetes it is.

Q **I am in my early twenties and have been diagnosed as diabetic. I am concerned that I will have to inject myself with insulin for the rest of my life. Is there no treatment to put an end to it?**

A Diabetes is not curable because it is due to a deficiency of insulin. However, it is an easily controlled condition. Although insulin injections make a tremendous difference to the daily life of a diabetic, the management of the condition is very much concerned as well with the essentials of everyday life, such as eating and exercise. So how much your life is affected is to a large degree within your control. Every country has excellent Diabetic Associations which will give you every support and any information you need.

Q My mother has just been told she has 'maturity onset' diabetes. She's not that old, only in her fifties, but I am not sure how she will cope with daily injections. Also I hadn't noticed any real change in her condition, should I have done?

A This is a form of diabetes that doesn't normally come on until middle or old age. It progresses very slowly and there are no dramatic attacks related to very high or low blood sugar. Often the patient will not be aware they have a problem at all until it is picked up by a doctor. Once her condition has been stabilized she will probably be maintained with diet alone, or diet with tablets. The long-term use of insulin injections is very rarely necessary with 'maturity onset' diabetes.

Q I understand that there are now self-test kits for diabetes. How do these work and how do I get hold of them?

A These kits are designed to help diabetics take their own blood sugar tests at home, so that visits to the doctor can be kept to a minimum. Only a drop of blood is needed, taken from either the finger or earlobe, using a disposable lancet. The test depends upon dipping an impregnated stick of chemicals into that one drop of blood. This will then change colour depending on the level of sugar. The colour is matched against standard colours provided, and a very quick result is obtained. These kits, and the disposable lancets, will be prescribed by the doctor so that diabetics can ensure that their levels of blood sugar are within a safe range.

Q **I have been a diabetic for many years and am well controlled on diet and tablets alone, but I still cannot lose all the weight my doctor would like me to. What else can I try?**

A It is important not to carry too much weight if you are diabetic because it may lead to complications later. If you have tried ordinary diets to no avail then perhaps a slimming club might be the answer. The encouragement of trying to lose weight with other people might be the spur you need. However, you must be particularly careful to use a balanced diet and make sure your doctor is happy with the one you've chosen.

Q **I am a diabetic and need daily injections of insulin. I am using disposable syringes and needles, but am concerned about how to get rid of them safely.**

A It's a very good point, because it is vital to dispose of them so they cannot fall into anyone else's hands. If you talk to your doctor s/he will be able to prescribe a clipping service which cuts off part of the needle and so makes it unusable in the future, if it is ever retrieved from your bin.

Q **I have heard that bran can help in the treatment of diabetes. How does this work?**

A A particular form of bran — guar — can modify the symptoms of those diabetics who only need diet or tablets to control their disease. Guar can help reduce the high blood sugar level this sort of diabetic experiences after a meal. It also reduces the blood fat levels that are common in this type of diabetes and which are responsible for a great number of the side effects and problems. Discuss it with your doctor before starting to take guar as it should be started slowly, say two and a half grams a day at first, and then gradually increased to five grams taken three times a day.

Q **My sister has been diagnosed as having cancer of the liver. The doctors have been marvellous in explaining everything, but I just feel I need to talk to someone else about it — about the non-medical side. Is there any organization that offers this service?**

A Most countries offer a service of this kind, usually run by those with personal experience of this problem. In the UK Dr Vicky Clement-Jones realized that there was a gap in cancer care when she herself was treated for cancer. She founded BACUP, the British Association of Cancer United Patients and their families and friends. Her work is carried on by BACUP who are always willing to lend an ear and offer what advice they can. You can reach them by telephone on 071 608 1661 between 10 am and 5.30 pm every weekday and up to 7 pm on Tuesdays and Thursdays.

Q **My mother has cancer which is now very advanced. She is taking lots of painkillers and the visiting nurse has suggested that she takes morphine by mouth. I am afraid of her becoming very sleepy and addicted to the drug. However long she is with us, I would like her to be as alert as possible.**

A Oral morphine is now given as the preferred medicine for patients with severe pain. The dose can be adjusted very easily so that your mother will get the maximum amount of pain relief without feeling dopey. The addictive properties of morphine are not important when you are treating patients with a relatively short lifespan, which unhappily your mother now has.

Q   **My mother is to have her spleen removed and she doesn't seem to want to talk about it. I can't ask her, but where is the spleen in the body, and what does it do?**

A   It is situated near the stomach, on the left, and is about the size of a fist. It has a consistency similar to liver and it's main function is to destroy old or deformed red blood cells. It also plays a very important part in providing resistance to infections.

Q   **My sister has anaemia and they suddenly decided to remove her spleen. I am worried because I believe that without a spleen she will not live as long as she would have done. Exactly what difference will it make?**

A   The spleen is usually removed as a treatment for severe forms of anaemia where it is breaking down too many red blood cells and causing jaundice. If the spleen becomes damaged or split open, as a result of an accident, then it is removed as a matter of urgency because it bleeds profusely when damaged. The absence of a spleen will certainly not shorten your sister's life.

Gallstones

Q   **What kind of people get gallstones?**

A   They are more likely to occur in women than in men, and are also more common in those who are overweight. As many as one in ten adults get gallstones, but the vast majority of them are entirely symptom-free.

Q **What are the symptoms of gallstones?**

A Chronic gallstones usually give pain or discomfort related to eating, and this is made worse by fatty meals. The pain tends to be concentrated under the right ribcage.

Q **I keep getting a very severe pain, just under my right ribcage. My urine has become quite dark in colour and my bowel motions are pale. What is causing this?**

A You must see your doctor for a thorough examination. It sounds like a gallstone is obstructing the duct which takes the bile from the gall bladder into the intestine. You may also be jaundiced, and this is caused by the yellow pigment of the bile getting back into the bloodstream.

Q **My doctor has diagnosed gallstones. What sort of treatment may be necessary?**

A There are two types of treatment available, provided there is no accompanying jaundice. Very tiny stones can be dissolved away by medicines containing bile acids and the doctor may make special dietary recommendations as well. If the stones are causing a real problem then surgical removal of the gallbladder and its stones (cholecystectomy) will be advised. Recently, it has proved possible to break down gallstones by sound waves — Lithotripsy.

Q **I would like to know what sort of scarring I will have after a gallbladder operation?**

A The scar is usually on the right side of the body. It will be about an inch or two below, and usually parallel to the lower ribcage or, alternatively, it will run up and down to the right of your navel. The scar will be about 6-8 inches long, depending on how fat you are.

Q **Is there anything I can do to prepare myself before going into hospital for a gallbladder operation?**

A Two things can help with all abdominal operations. First, make sure that you are not overweight at all. Second, if you are a smoker you should give it up at least a month before you go into hospital.

Glands

Q **Where is the thyroid gland located in the body?**

A It is in the neck and is a small gland with two lobes lying each side of the voice box.

Q **Why is the thyroid so important to us?**

A The thyroid is very important because it makes the hormone thyroxine. This is responsible for helping us to grow properly and for developing our intelligence. Once we become adult, the thyroid hormone enables us to use our food to maintain our good health.

Q **I am very overweight and nothing I do seems to shift it. Do I have an underactive thyroid?**

A It is very rare for obesity to be a symptom of thyroid deficiency, but if you think you are an exception then it can be very quickly checked out by your doctor with a simple blood test.

Q **I have cancer of the thyroid, but it took some time to diagnose. Why was this?**

A Thyroid cancer is not very common. It usually comes on painlessly as an unequal swelling of the neck and it is difficult to differentiate between a cancer and simple cyst. Ultrasound or CT scan shows whether a lump is solid or cystic, and scanning with radioactive iodine may show 'hot spots' associated with possible cancer.

Q **How is cancer of the thyroid dealt with?**

A Treatment is usually surgical removal of either one lobe or the whole thyroid; the patient then takes thyroid hormone replacement tablets for the rest of his or her life.

Q **I have just come out of hospital after an operation on my thyroid. I have got a large scar around my throat which I am told will get fainter in time. Should I put any cream on to keep the scar and surrounding area supple?**

A The scar must look very unsightly to you right now, but it will become much, much fainter. In fact after one or two years it's often difficult to see a thyroid scar at all. The skin around the neck is well supplied with blood vessels and the scar heals quickly. It is not necessary to put any cream on it, but some people find that vitamins E and C, taken by mouth, can help to heal wounds more rapidly.

Q My mother has just been diagnosed as having myxoedema. I can't really see any change in her condition, and I am very upset that none of us noticed she was becoming ill. What should we have been looking for?

A Please don't blame yourself for this. It is an illness that can be very difficult to spot because it comes on so slowly. What happens is that the thyroid very gradually stops working and the changes involved are so subtle that even the patient's regular doctor cannot always guarantee to pick it up. The symptoms are forgetfulness; loss of hair on the head and eyebrows; thickening of the skin; a perpetual feeling of cold, and a very slow pulse rate in someone who is not at all athletic.

Q My sister has been told she has to have an operation for Graves' Disease. We thought at first it was cancer because she lost so much weight. Will the operation completely cure her?

A Graves' Disease, or overactive thyroid, is usually first treated by giving a course of tablets. The sufferer has a ravenous appetite but loses weight, chatters away continually and may also have shaking hands and staring, wide-open, prominent eyes. If it is not possible to regulate the illness with tablets, then it is usual to remove part of the thyroid gland in order to bring it back to a normal level of production. Like all the hormone glands, the thyroid is very complex, but the operation should bring the condition under control. Your sister will need regular monitoring in the future to make sure her thyroid doesn't go underactive.

Q   **I have an unsightly goitre in my neck. Will it go down again of its own accord or should I get some treatment for it?**

A   Goitre can be caused by lack of iodine in the diet and remedying this may go some way towards helping. Unfortunately this swelling of the thyroid does not respond to hormone tablets and may have to be removed surgically. The swelling could also be due to cysts or other growths so it is important to have it checked by your doctor.

Teeth, bones and muscles

The whole structure of our body depends upon us having a strong skeletal framework of bones to support us. Connected to the bones, cartilages or ligaments are the muscles which contract in response to messages from the brain and give us the power of movement. Strong, healthy teeth are developed through proper care in childhood and are essential to prepare our food for digestion.

Teeth

Q   **How many teeth should we have if we have never had any taken out?**

A   For the normal adult that would be a total of 32 teeth. Four of these are wisdom teeth and may not always come through the gum to be visible in the mouth.

Q   **On the chart the dentist makes of my teeth I notice they have different names. What do they mean?**

A   There are four different types of tooth and they have different actions to deal with food. Cutting and biting actions are done by the incisors and canines at the front, and the chewing by the premolars and molars at the back.

Q **What is the proper way to clean teeth?**

A When we brush our teeth it is the junction between the gums and the teeth which should be cleaned, not just the surface of the tooth. Use a soft, anti-plaque brush and toothpaste and go right over every tooth with a circular motion. Then gently press the bristles up into any gap between the gums and the tooth and rotate the brush in a circular way, with a press and roll action, to clean out any food debris before it becomes plaque.

Q **What causes toothache?**

A In the middle of each tooth is an area called the pulp. It contains the blood vessels which nourish the teeth and nerve fibres which are very sensitive to heat, cold, pressure and pain. If you have any decay in a tooth, even a tiny cavity, then bacteria can pass through to the pulp. This becomes infected and the swollen tissues give rise to pain — toothache.

Q **How would I know if the pulp in my tooth was inflamed?**

A You generally get an ache in that tooth. Usually eating very hot, cold, or sweet things will trigger it off.

Q **How common is it to have false teeth?**

A In the UK around 30 per cent of people no longer have their own teeth. In the USA the figure is much lower, at around 14 per cent.

Q **What do healthy gums look like?**

A They're usually pale pink, or brown, in colour
(depending on your racial type) and look firm.
They won't bleed when you clean them, and they
cling to the teeth smoothly.

Q **What's the reason for using dental floss?**

A It's a good way of removing plaque and food
particles that can remain between the teeth after
eating.

Q **I know it's a good idea to use dental floss, but
I'm not sure exactly what to do with it?**

A You need to take about 18 inches (500mm) of
floss and secure each end by winding it around
the first or second fingers on each hand. You
insert the floss in the gap between two teeth and
then using a gentle, sawing, motion draw the floss
backwards and forwards between the teeth.

Q **I go to the dentist regularly to have my teeth
scaled and my gums always bleed. Is this
usual?**

A To do its job properly, the instrument used for
scaling has to get right down to the base of the
tooth. This may cause some gum bleeding, which
is quite a normal reaction.

Q I would like to have some of my teeth replaced as they are very discoloured. How long does it take to have crowns fitted?

A It usually takes two to three visits. On the first the dentist will discuss what you want and prepare the tooth ready for the crown to be fitted. When the crown has been made you go back and the dentist will fit it into place.

Q What happens after the dentist has drilled the tooth away ready for the crown? Do you go about like that until the crown is ready?

A No, the dentist will fit a temporary crown so that you can eat normally, and not look too different from usual.

Q What are crowns made of?

A If it's a tooth that is usually seen, such as in the front of your mouth, then it is usually made of white porcelain. The back teeth need a stronger material for all the chewing that they have to do, so teeth for that area are usually crowned using gold or a gold and platinum alloy.

Q My teeth seem to have become rather discoloured recently. What can have caused it?

A It could be a number of things. Smoking, certain drugs, the effects of ageing can all leave their mark on your teeth. Also, if you have a tooth that has died, then it will tend to have a rather grey appearance.

Q **My daughter had an impacted wisdom tooth that gave her a lot of trouble. What does 'impacted' mean?**

A It means that it has become trapped by the tooth next to it so that it fails to emerge properly from the gum.

Q **Why do wisdom teeth give so much trouble?**

A During human development over many thousands of years our jaws have become slightly smaller. Wisdom teeth are the last to grow and you may find there isn't enough room in the jawbone for them. So they come out sideways, pushing into the tooth in front, or give a lot of pain while they are trying to come through.

Q **I have had a lot of problems with my wisdom teeth, and so did my mother. You can't inherit tooth problems can you?**

A Problems with wisdom teeth do seem to run in families. You may have inherited the same shape of jaw as your mother, so you will have the same type of problems as she did.

Q **Where did wisdom teeth get their name?**

A Wisdom teeth are so named because they appear between the ages of 18 and 25, by which time we *should* have gained our wisdom!

Q **Is it true that eating sweets is the main reason why we lose teeth?**

A Sugar is certainly very bad indeed for your teeth, but the main reason that adults lose teeth is not from tooth decay, but gum disease.

Q **What is plaque?**

A Plaque is the scraps of food and other debris in the mouth which get coated with calcium salts, making it tough and brittle.

Q **Why does plaque cause so much trouble?**

A Deposits of plaque build up between the tooth and the gum and these deposits gradually force the gum away from the tooth. The separated gum becomes thickened and reddened and is susceptible to infection from the many millions of bacteria which live in our mouths. As the gum is forced away from the tooth, the delicate bone of the tooth socket becomes reabsorbed and the socket shallower, eventually making the tooth loose.

Q **What is gingivitis?**

A It means infection of the gums. Often it's caused by plaque forming at the base of the teeth. This irritates the gums and they become infected and swollen. The gums bleed very easily and look red and swollen.

Q **Is gingivitis very common?**

A In a mild form, probably nine out of ten adults will get it at some time.

Q **Is anyone particularly prone to gingivitis?**

A It seems that if you are diabetic or expecting a baby then you are more likely to get gingivitis.

Bones

Q **My friend was in a car crash and had a broken back. Within two weeks she was walking around as usual. I thought if you broke your back you were paralysed?**

A It depends on where the injury occurred and exactly what was damaged. The spine encloses the spinal cord, the nervous tissue which carries all the messages between the brain and the limbs and trunk. If just the bones of the spine were damaged, and the spinal cord is merely bruised or squashed, then the back will probably return to normal functioning in a short time. If, however, the damaged bones cross each other and injure the spinal cord, then paralysis will occur.

Q **Since I was paralysed after a fall last year I have had excellent treatment but think more could be done to help us once we have left hospital. Is there an organization that does this?**

A Many countries have self-help groups to cover this situation. In the UK, the Spinal Injuries Association was founded in 1974 and is an organization for paralysed people, their friends and families. It is a clearing house for all information about spinal injuries and acts as a pressure group to improve the lot of sufferers.

Q Last year my daughter was injured in a motorbike crash. Her neck was broken, she cannot move her arms or legs, and is now confined to a wheelchair. We have done everything we can to help her, but money is now getting tight. Is there anywhere to go for help?

A In 1988 the Independent Living Fund was created in the UK to assist very disabled people who need paid domestic help or personal care if they are to live in their own homes. Your local DHSS office will give you all the details you need to apply to this fund.

Q My new job is in a shop and I have to move stock around in boxes. I have started to get a lot of back pain. I don't want to give up my job so is there anything I can do about my back?

A The most helpful thing to learn is how to lift things properly with the least strain on your back. First, always test the heaviness of a load *before* you lift it and get help if necessary. Next, always bend your knees when lifting and keep your back straight so that your legs are doing the work, not your back. Finally, don't try and lift things wearing high heels because that is just putting more strain on your back.

Q What causes back pain?

A The back is a very complicated piece of engineering. There are 24 independent moving vertebrae between your skull and your hip, and each one has over six moving joints. Each joint is closely associated with a network of nerve endings and if you put pressure on any one of them then it can give rise to excruciating pain.

Q **What is the usual cause of back pain?**

A The most common cause of back pain is torn ligaments or muscle fibres due to strain. This is very common when either lifting something incorrectly or trying to lift something that is too heavy.

Q **What is ankylosing spondylitis?**

A Spondylitis refers to an inflammation of the joints which link our separate backbones into the flexible spinal column. Ankylosing means that as a result of this inflammation the small joints around the spinal column are destroyed and replaced by bone which effectively splints or fixes the spinal column. If enough of these small joints are affected then mobility of the neck and trunk is greatly diminished. The spine then becomes stiff and, unless great care is taken, it may fix in a bent rather than a straight position.

Q **What causes ankylosing spondylitis?**

A It is not known what causes this condition but it is much more common in men than women, in a ratio of eight to one. One in every 2000 people is affected and there does seem to be a tendency for it to be inherited. People with a particular blood type (HLA 27) are much more at risk than others.

Q **I have had back pain on and off for a few months and a friend has suggested seeing a chiropractor. What do they do?**

A Back pain is an area where preventative and alternative medicine can make a good contribution. Chiropractors specialize in the diagnosis and treatment of mechanical disorders of the spine. Discuss this with your doctor.

Q **I have been taking painkillers for a pain in my hip joint but would like to try to do without them. Would going to an osteopath be any help?**

A Osteopathy is a manipulative therapy which uses massage and spinal manipulation and many people have found relief from similar problems to yours by consulting an osteopath. Talk to your doctor about it before you make a decision.

Q **How can I be sure that I get a good osteopath?**

A Word of mouth is often a good guide and your doctor may well be able to suggest someone locally. There are usually national registers for alternative therapists and your local library should be able to put you in touch with them.

Q **What is the Alexander Technique? A friend says it has cured her back problem.**

A It is a system that was founded by an Australian, Mr F. M. Alexander, in order to correct the misuse and abuse of the skeleton through years of slouching, slumping, tensing up and general bad posture. You will need to go to a registered teacher who will identify your particular problem and then work with you to correct it through a series of rehabilitation and re-educative exercises. It is a very gentle way of identifying the root of many of our physical and non-physical ailments.

Q **I fractured my shoulder quite badly in an accident some time ago and it still gives me a lot of trouble. Why is it taking so long to get better?**

A Shoulders are very troublesome joints when they are injured. The shoulder is the most mobile joint in the whole body and any damage or restriction of movement is likely to give rise to adhesions within the joint capsule which are very painful to break down.

Q **Will any sort of exercise help with a shoulder injury?**

A Swimming or exercising your shoulder in water regularly will help a lot, especially in the early days after an injury. An osteopath might also be able to get some mobility back into the joint.

Q **What is a compound fracture?**

A Compound means that the ends of the broken bone are open to the outside world through a cut in the skin. Even a graze over a fracture can make it compound; you don't need to actually be able to see the bone sticking through the skin. They are usually treated with antibiotics, and anti-tetanus protection is also important.

Q **If you break a leg why do they put it in traction?**

A Fracture of the leg bones often give trouble because the muscles around the bones are so strong that they continually pull the bone out of shape. Traction has to be applied continuously to counteract this muscle pull and it has to be delicately balanced so that the ends of the bone are not pulled apart but rest together.

Q Is there an alternative to traction for a broken leg? Surely there must be a better way of helping it to mend?

A Traction can get rather tedious so, in some people, an operation is carried out. This consists of either driving a rod down the centre of the bone, or screwing a metal plate onto the outside of the bone to fix the ends together.

Q Over the years my sister and I have both had various accidents of one kind or another, but she always seems to heal so much quicker than I do. Why is this?

A Unfortunately people and their bones are not the same — even when it is in one family. Some heal quickly and some more slowly. Broken bones have to be immobilized or treated until the broken ends have knit back together. This may be six to ten weeks, or six months — you can only heal at your own pace.

Q My doctor has told me I have osteoporosis — what exactly does this mean?

A Osteoporosis means thinning of the bones. Bones are made up of fibrous tissue into which hard calcium salts are deposited to give them strength. In osteoporosis the calcium part of the bone becomes less strong and the bones tend to collapse. This is a very gradual process, but it is the reason why many women (and men) tend to lose height as they get older. In more severe cases the bones become fragile, to the extent that they break after even a modest tumble.

Q **I am worried about osteoporosis. Does it happen to every women after the menopause?**

A No, not at all. A great deal depends on the general level of calcium in the body. It is important that good calcium levels are maintained throughout the adult life and particularly during and after the menopause.

Q **I've heard that exercise is a good thing to prevent osteoporosis. Is this true?**

A Exercise is a very important bone protector. It keeps the muscles strong and active and this keeps the bones 'fit' too.

Q **How does a lack of calcium cause osteoporosis?**

A Calcium deficiency is a very rare cause of osteoporosis in healthy adults. However, the problem is that the body has very specific daily requirements of calcium. Certain quantities are forcibly excreted by us every day whether we are taking enough of it in our food or not. It is when we do not have enough calcium in our diet that the extra is pulled out of our bones to make up the deficit. In the bones, calcium is responsible for maintaining the rigid structure, so the loss of calcium gives rise to thinning of the bones.

Q **How much calcium do I need every day?**

A The daily requirement is probably about 500 mg a day, but to be on the safe side the Australian Nutrition Council advises an intake of about 800 mg a day. You would get that in about a pint of milk, or a couple of calcium tablets, and it doesn't matter whether the milk is skimmed or not, the calcium content is the same. Cheese, milk, bread and cereals are all good sources of calcium.

Q **On a recent skiing holiday I fell quite hard on my right shoulder. It was OK at the time but when I got back it began to be very painful. I saw the doctor and she said it was a 'frozen' shoulder. Is it a type of skiing injury?**

A No, a 'frozen' shoulder just refers to the fact that the joint is very painful to move so you tend to 'freeze' it motionless to avoid discomfort. Any kind of damage or strain can cause a disturbance to the complex system of muscles and tendons playing over the shoulder, whether it is skiing or just over-exertion.

Q **I injured my shoulder muscles playing tennis last summer and was surprised to be told to keep the joint moving. Doesn't it need rest to get better?**

A It is sensible to protect the shoulder and restrict movement for the day or so of acute pain that follows just after the injury. After that you should take painkillers as needed and start to exercise the joint, but without weight bearing on it. If it is left to rest it quickly builds up fibrous scar tissue which restricts the movements further and makes it even more painful to get back to normal.

Q **What is good exercise for stiff joints?**

A Swimming is an excellent all-round form of exercise because all joint movements are so much easier to do in water, and the joints don't have to bear the weight of the body.

Q **My mother has severe arthritis in her hands. What exactly has caused it?**

A There are many different forms of this disease and by far the most common is osteoarthritis which is due to 'fair wear and tear'. Where bones meet other bones to form a moving joint there is a protective covering of cartilage or gristle over the surface of the bone which stops them wearing away. After injury, or simply as the result of use during a long life, the cartilage may become worn away and the joints become stiff and painful to move.

Q **My daughter was struck down with arthritis when she was only 11 years old. This has left her quite disabled, but she is a great fighter and holds down a good job in computing. She is having a very serious relationship with a man and I am very worried about whether she can possibly cope with family life.**

A As she has done so well in coming to terms with her life so far, it would seem only reasonable to suppose that she will be able to carry on doing so. It would seem very unfair to deny her the chance of married life and all that it implies. Why not discuss your worries openly with her. She knows how much you care for her.

Q **My mother has arthritis, but she refuses to believe what the doctor tells her and doesn't take the tablets she has been given. Why is she behaving like this?**

A This is not so uncommon as you might think. Coming to terms with the diagnosis of arthritis is not always easy. For many people it seems simply a sign of increasing age, which they resist with vigour. Others fear that such a diagnosis means that they will eventually be helpless cripples and, not surprisingly, they don't want to admit such a terrible possibility. Reassure your mother that arthritis is not a sign of ageing, it can affect young as well as old, and that the vast majority of sufferers remain quite independent.

Q **I had what I thought was an inflamed shoulder joint — it was painful and swollen — but my doctor says I have rheumatoid arthritis. The shoulder is back to normal now, so surely it can't have been arthritis?**

A Rheumatoid arthritis normally starts as an acute condition with all the hallmarks of inflammation. The affected joints are painful, hot, red, swollen and difficult to move. The sufferer usually feels 'under the weather' too and there may be a low-grade fever. This type of arthritis can run a short sharp course and can disappear almost as quickly as it came, and you were fortunate that this is what happened in your case.

Q **What happens in a severe case of rheumatoid arthritis?**

A It can be a very prolonged and protracted disease. When the painful phase of the illness has passed the joints may be left very distorted and the muscles severely wasted by months of disuse.

Q Is there any diet which can help, or prevent, arthritis?

A Arthritis is not just one single disease, it is a whole variety of conditions, so it is difficult to say whether purely dietary measures can either help or prevent it. There are two diet supplements which have proved useful in some cases of arthritis; they are pure cod liver oil and extract of the green-lipped mussel, both obtainable from health food shops or chemists. An alternative practitioner such as a naturopath or homoeopath might have some recommendations on diet for you, or you could read one of the many specialist books on the subject.

Q I have read about specialist diets being recommended for arthritis. What do they consist of?

A Most diets for this condition usually suggest cutting out red meat, alcohol, sugar and refined or processed foods. There are plenty of goods books on specialist diets for arthritis, your local health store will be able to advise you.

Q I have been on medicine for my arthritis for a few years now, but it still seems to upset my stomach. Can I do anything about it?

A Many of the medicines used to treat arthritis have side-effects on the stomach. They can cause tiny gastric ulcers which can be a source of great discomfort. As you have been on your present medicine for some time, it would be sensible to talk to your doctor and see whether changing to a new prescription might not benefit you.

Q **I have been taking aspirin for my arthritis for the last year but am worried about newspaper reports which claim aspirin causes stomach ulcers. What should I do?**

A Drugs to combat arthritis are known as Non-Steroidal Anti-Inflammatory Drugs, or NSAIDs for short. Aspirin is the best known of these and most of the side-effects you have seen described can be avoided by taking the drugs in the proper way. Always take them with food or immediately after a meal, never on an empty stomach. When you take the tablets stand up so they go straight down to the stomach and there is no risk of them settling in the oesophagus and causing irritation there. If you take soluble aspirin then you reduce the chance of this even more.

Q **What exactly is gout?**

A Gout is a rarer form of arthritis and occurs when the body is unable to deal with a chemical called uric acid. This is a normal compound which we all make and is cleared out of the body by the kidneys. Sufferers have too much uric acid in their blood and it is then deposited as crystals within the joints. This is what causes the inflammation and pain of gout.

Q **My father and one of my aunts suffered greatly from gout. Am I likely to get it too?**

A It is very much an inherited disease due to a chemical defect, but it is more common in men than women. A simple blood test will establish if you also have gout.

Q **Is there anything I can do to prevent an attack of gout?**

A An attack can often be precipitated in a susceptible person by overloading the system with foods which contain high levels of uric acid, such as fish roe or large quantities of port or claret. Paradoxically starvation can also bring on an attack, so extreme diets should be avoided.

Q **What are bunions?**

A A bunion is an inflamed collection of fluid at the side of the great toe where it joins onto the foot proper.

Q **Does anything in particular cause bunions?**

A It is nearly always associated with the turning-in of the great toes which is often the result of wearing shoes that are too small, or continued use of high heels.

Q **My mother has terrible bunions. What can I do to avoid getting them?**

A Generally bunions can be prevented by keeping the foot properly exercised and wearing sensible shoes.

Q **Do bunions always need treatment?**

A For many sufferers the only problem is an unsightly distortion which can cause some difficulty in walking and make buying shoes more tricky than usual. This is known as Hallus Valgus. In these cases no medical treatment is required.

Q **I have a very painful bunion. What can I do about it?**

A If a bunion becomes very inflamed then it needs treatment by antibiotics to cure the infection.

Q **My bunions seem to be getting worse and I don't want to keep taking antibiotics. What other treatment is there?**

A If acute episodes keep recurring, or the deformity becomes worse, then an operation may be necessary.

Q **Is it quite a straightforward surgical procedure to operate on bunions?**

A The procedure itself is straightforward, but it is not always an easy operation. It can be extremely painful, may lead to difficulty in walking and can take a long time to heal.

Q **If I have my bunions operated on does that mean I will never have any more trouble from them?**

A Unfortunately, no. There are a few cases where, even after surgery, the bunions recur. It is believed that this is due to the way that you walk, and the distribution of weight over your feet.

Q **I am going to have my bunions treated soon. I never feel dressed unless I am wearing high heels and am worried that the operation may stop me from wearing them.**

A The only person who can really give you the answer is the surgeon who is carrying out the operation. In any event, the bones take some time to heal and you may not be comfortable in anything other than flat shoes for quite a while.

Q I think I might have ingrowing toenails. Just what do they look like?

A An ingrowing toenail occurs when the nail of any toe curves under at the sides, biting into the flesh. The great toe is the most commonly affected.

Q Is there anything that can be done about an ingrowing toenail?

A If you think you have an ingrowing toenail, then consult either your doctor or a chiropodist. If necessary they may recommend a small operation to remove the edge of the nail and the nail fold which produces it.

Q I have now had two ingrowing toenails. How can I make sure I don't get any more?

A To stop the condition recurring you should wear well-fitting shoes and ensure that the area round your big toe nail is kept clean and dry. When you cut your toenails make sure that the nail is cut straight across the top and that no splinters are left at the edge.

Q I am going to have my arm in plaster for a couple of months and I am worried about getting in and out of the bath.

A Have a hand rail put up so you can grab it for support to ease yourself in and out of the bath. Make sure it is very securely fixed and can withstand your full weight.

Q How do I stop the plaster on my arm getting wet when I have a bath?

A Rig up an old roller towel attached to your shower rail. You can then rest your elbow and forearm in this cradle while you are in the bath.

Cosmetic surgery

Q **I am 17 and recently broke my nose in an accident. It is now very ugly and I would like to have it operated on.**

A You will need to see a specialist — either a plastic surgeon or a specialist in facio-maxillary work. S/he will then decide the best time to operate on you.

Q **I have decided to have my nose shape altered. How do I go about it?**

A This procedure is known as rhinoplasty and it is not something to undertake lightly. You should think very carefully about why you are having this operation. Discuss it with your doctor first, and if you then decide to proceed you should make it quite clear to your chosen surgeon what you want from this procedure, both physically and psychologically. Do remember that surgical operations do not always give perfect results.

Q **Just what will the operation on my nose involve?**

A The cartilage of the nose is reshaped during the operation into the shape you want. Only very rarely is it necessary to alter the tiny nasal bones which join the nose to the skull.

Q **My friend has just had her nose altered and I can't see any scarring at all. How is this done?**

A The scars are inside the nose so that nothing is visible when the wound has healed.

Q **Will I be given a general or a local anaesthetic when I have my nose operated on?**

A It will depend entirely on the extent of the operation and your general health. If there is not too much work to be done then you will probably be given a local anaesthetic. Your surgeon should discuss this with you when s/he outlines the details of your particular operation.

Q **What happens after a nose operation?**

A Immediately afterwards the nose is packed with gauze and you may have a plaster cast or splint put on. This is to prevent any movement while the nose is healing. This should take about ten days. For three weeks afterwards you must not blow your nose and you might find that it is numb for a couple of months. Usually within six months you should be fully recovered.

Q **What will I look like after the operation?**

A There is usually quite a lot of swelling and bruising underneath your eyes and this can look quite startling. Your nose will also be very sore.

Muscles

Q **I think I have got housemaid's knee. It's quite painful and swollen. What has caused it?**

A Housemaid's knee and tennis elbow are common names for bursitis. Where tendons run over bones, such as the knee or elbow joints, there are often sacs of fluid or bursas. Their purpose is to reduce friction to a minimum, but occasionally these sacs of fluid become inflamed or irritated: they then swell up and contain excess fluid.

Q **What's the usual treatment for bursitis?**

A Simple treatment starts by binding with a support bandage, thus reducing the amount of work done by that particular joint. Usually this is enough to control the swelling and it then subsides of its own accord.

Q **I have had tennis elbow for a couple of weeks now but it doesn't seem to be getting better. What do I do now?**

A If the problem lasts longer than two to three weeks you should go back to see your doctor. S/he may suggest that you undergo injection treatment combined with drainage of the distended sac.

Q **What exactly is a hernia?**

A Hernia simply means a protrusion or bulge. It usually occurs in the abdomen and is made by a pocket of the peritoneum, which is a delicate membrane lining the abdomen. This pocket can also contain loops of intestine.

Q **Do women suffer from hernias at all?**

A There are many different types of hernia but the most common is the type found in the groin (inguinal hernia), and certainly men suffer more from this than women do. However, women are just as prone to the other types such as hiatus and umbilical hernias.

Q **I have got a para-umbilical hernia. Will I need an operation?**

A This type of hernia occurs for the first time in adults and is more common in women than men. It can cause problems and repair by operation is usually advised.

Q **I have a small hernia that the doctor has advised me to have operated on. I'm not sure what this involves, but wouldn't it be better to wait until it gives me real discomfort?**

A The operation consists of repairing the damaged hole in the muscles. It is much better carried out while the weakness in the muscle is still small. The surgical treatment of major hernias is designed to relieve the discomfort of the bulge and prevent strangulation of the gut.

Q **How long will I have to go into hospital for a hernia operation?**

A It will depend on the type of hernia you have, but many of these operations can be carried out on a day-care basis and you can then convalesce in the comfort of your own home. Do discuss this with your surgeon.

Q **I have recently been suffering from pain and numbness in my hands and have been told I have Carpal Tunnel Syndrome. Can you explain this to me?**

A This occurs when one of the main nerves to the hand is compressed. The carpal tunnel is a tiny gap on the front of the tightly bound muscle tendons which run from the forearm into the hand. Any swelling of the tissues in this area may cause compression of the nerve.

Q How do you get Carpal Tunnel Syndrome?

A It can occur temporarily during pregnancy and more permanently in cases of arthritis.

Q Is there anything I can do about Carpal Tunnel Syndrome?

A Treatment includes taking diuretics to get rid of the excess fluid, and splinting the wrist at night to stop excessive bending. If these measures do not work then an operation may be necessary.

Q My daughter is a tennis fanatic but has been having trouble with her knee. The doctor says it is cartilage trouble. Just what is cartilage?

A Cartilage problems are the bane of many athletes' lives. Wherever two bones move together in a joint the surfaces are covered by cartilage. The surfaces of the thigh bone (femur) and one of the leg bones (tibia), which form the knee joint, are so different in shape that two extra bits of cartilage are built into the system to help adjust the surfaces to each other. These half-moon-shaped discs of cartilage are very vulnerable to damage in the hurly burly of active sport.

Q Will my damaged cartilage heal on its own?

A Sometimes they heal with rest. Often one or the other will become so damaged that it will need to be removed by surgery. Your doctor will advise you if that becomes necessary.

Q **My daughter recently sprained her ankle at work and when she was sent home I didn't know what to do for her. What is the correct treatment for a sprain?**

A The immediate treatment for a sprain or strain is to prevent the swelling and bruising that accompanies it. If you apply an ice pack immediately this will stop all the bruising and swelling. Then if you can sleep with an ice pack on the sprain, the next morning you will find the joint much more comfortable and easy to use. After the first 24 hours a good protective crepe bandage or plaster strapping is all that is usually required to keep the sprain at bay.

Q **I have a couple of crepe bandages in my first aid box, but they seem very loose. Will they be any good for bandaging?**

A Crepe bandages should be rinsed through regularly in warm soapy water to retain their elasticity.

Q **Where is the Achilles tendon?**

A It is probably the strongest tendon in the whole body and it joins the calf muscles to the back of the heel bone.

Q **If the Achilles tendon is ruptured, what happens?**

A The immediate effect of a rupture is that you lose ankle power. You can't walk very easily because you can't push off on your toes.

Q **How is a ruptured tendon treated?**

A Unfortunately tendons heal very badly. They have few blood vessels, so don't heal well without help. The ends of the ruptured tendons may have sprung anything up to two or three inches apart. This means that the tendon has to be sewn together in a surgical operation. Then the knee and ankle joints must be immobilized so that no tension goes on to the heel and tendon, this usually means up to six weeks in plaster.

Q **I have a silly problem that comes on if I have to sit still for long periods. My legs get so fidgety and uncomfortable that I try and avoid going anywhere where I can't get up and move around. Is there really anything wrong with me?**

A This condition was first described as far back as 1685 and is commonly known as 'restless legs'. The most general symptom is an unpleasant creeping sensation deep in the legs that comes on particularly in the evenings. There is a compulsion to move around when these sensations start and just one or both legs can be affected.

Q **What causes 'restless legs' to start?**

A There is no known cause but it seems to be more common during pregnancy and in people with anaemia or rheumatoid arthritis. Similar symptoms to these do occur as a side-effect of certain drugs, but in this case the sensation persists throughout the day and immediately improves when the medication stops.

Q **Is there any treatment for 'restless legs'?**

A Walking, massaging or rubbing the legs vigorously usually brings some relief but there is no real treatment that has been shown to be effective in controlling it.

Q **My mother and my aunt both suffer from lumbago, but they don't seem to have the same sort of pains. Just what does lumbago mean?**

A Lumbago can be due to many different causes. The name simply describes pain in the lower part of the back around the lumbar spine.

Q **Every time I attack the garden I end up with backache. What's the best thing to do for this?**

A First stop attacking the garden and take it more gently. It's the violent activity that is causing your muscles to protest. Little and often would be better than a marathon session once a week. Usually a couple of aspirin, a hot bath and some rest are all that's needed to cure this type of attack.

Q **A year ago I suffered a severe attack of pain in my back which the doctor said was lumbago. I have had another attack since and I want to know how I got it?**

A It can be brought on by too much unaccustomed activity, such as digging over the garden or moving all the furniture around. More seriously, it can also be due to a slipped disc or, very rarely, to actual bone disease. If you can find out exactly what is causing your lumbago then you will know how best to cope with it.

Q **One of my friends has just been told that she has Charcot Marie Tooth Disease. I've never heard of it before, is it quite rare?**

A It is an inherited condition which affects the nerves supplying certain muscles, especially those in the legs. It is an extremely rare and debilitating condition and its name comes simply from the people who first described the condition.

Q **Is there anyone who can give me advice about dealing with Charcot Marie Tooth Disease?**

A There is an international group which helps sufferers both to understand and manage their disease. Their address can be found in the Information Register.

Q **I have recently started getting pains in my calves when I walk to the shops. If I rest for a while the pain goes off.**

A It sounds like a condition called intermittent claudication. This occurs when the blood supply to the muscles in your legs has become inadequate to sustain active exercise. It is very important that you talk to your doctor, who will advise you as to what treatment is necessary.

Q **What causes intermittent claudication to occur?**

A Waste products build up in the muscles and because they are not washed away quickly enough they cause a great deal of pain. Obviously the pain passes off when you rest and reduce the amount of work that your muscles are doing.

Q **Will anything make intermittent claudication worse?**

A If you smoke this will probably aggravate the condition. High blood fat levels may also increase the deposits on the blood vessel walls which are causing them to narrow. Hence the problem.

Eyes and ears

Eyesight and the ability to distinguish sound are two of our most vital senses. It is through them that we form impressions of the world around us and, through our eyes, give out a potent indicator of our physical and emotional health.

Eyes

Q **I have just had a bout of conjunctivitis — how can I stop it happening again?**

A When you have conjunctivitis the delicate lining which covers the outer part of the eye and the eyelid becomes inflamed. Usually this is due to bacteria or viruses which can enter the eye if it is rubbed with dirty hands or a handkerchief. If you can avoid doing this it will be a great help. Occasionally, conjunctivitis can be due to allergies or can happen if you've been in an irritating atmosphere, like a very smoky room. It is better if your doctor sees you when you are in the middle of an attack so that a proper diagnosis and prescription can be given.

Q **What exactly are cataracts?**

A It is the name of a medical condition involving gradual loss of vision. Things appear misty, as if seen through a cataract of water, hence the name.

Q How are cataracts formed?

A There is a change in the chemical structure in the lens of the eye. Instead of being completely clear, parts of it become crystallized and don't let the light through properly. It can occur in the centre of the lens, where it will be more obvious, or around the edges where it can cause hardly any problems at all.

Q How long do cataracts take to form, and can they be prevented?

A There are no rules which govern the progress of a cataract, nor is there any known way of preventing it. Changes in the lens can progress very slowly and a lot of people with cataracts will never have a serious enough problem to need an operation. It is important, though, to have regular check-ups by an opthalmic surgeon as soon as you have been diagnosed as having cataracts.

Q We have just discovered that my mother has glaucoma. What is it and how will it affect her?

A Glaucoma is caused by a blockage which stops the eyeball fluid draining away, which it needs to do to maintain a normal pressure. If the pressure inside the eyeball goes up too high it can damage the retina. This happens very gradually and if only one eye is affected then the other will compensate for the vision loss. Many people are therefore not aware that they have glaucoma. This is why regular eye tests are very important, especially for the elderly.

Q In my left eye I keep having a sort of flittering zig-zag effect, in a red glow. It lasts about 20 minutes or so and I can't see for that time. I am just over 60 and wonder if it has to do with my age?

A It sounds as though you may have glaucoma. It does get more common in the elderly and is worse at night when the lights are dimmed. It needs to be treated as quickly as possible before your eyes suffer any more damage. Do see your optician as soon as possible.

Q What treatment is there for glaucoma?

A It can be treated simply by eye drops. Surgery is only used when medical treatments have failed, or if you find it impossible to use drops regularly.

Q Is glaucoma hereditary?

A There is a greater risk of becoming a glaucoma sufferer if someone in the family has it. Diabetics are also three times more likely to get it than non-diabetics. The sooner it is diagnosed the less likely you are to suffer from permanent loss of vision so it pays to have regular eye checks.

Q Recently I have had a problem with one of my eyes. The whole eyeball seems to move from side to side and I cannot focus properly. What should I do?

A It is possible that you are suffering from a condition called nystagmus and you should visit your doctor to discuss it. There are many causes of nystagmus and you will need special tests to find out exactly what the problem is.

Q I have been diagnosed as having retinitis pigmentosa and been told I will go totally blind over the next few years. I have not been offered any treatment, but is there anywhere I can go for some help and advice?

A This is an inherited condition and, unfortunately, at the moment there is no known cure or any way of halting the disease. However, research is going on and in the UK one fellow sufferer has set up the Retinitis Pigmentosa Society. There is a voluntary helpline on 0327 53276 which is available from 9am to 3pm and 6pm to 10pm each weekday.

Q When I was younger I had a form of cancer in my eye (retinoblastoma) and although it was treated successfully I was told it could affect any children I might have. What can I do?

A This type of cancer usually shows itself in young children, normally before they go to school. As you have discovered, it can be successfully cured but the condition is inherited. It is associated with low levels of a particular enzyme and when you are pregnant it is possible to have your unborn baby checked to see if it is carrying this cancer. The test is not generally available so you may need to ask your doctor to arrange it for you.

Q For some reason, one of my eyes has started flickering. What makes it do that?

A The muscles around the eye contract because of a simple muscle spasm. It can be irritating, but is nothing to worry about.

Q **I keep getting this black spot in front of one eye. I am 52 and wonder if it is just a sign of ageing?**

A Black spots — or floaters — are caused by blood cells which have been trapped in the fluid which fills the eyeball. Although floaters are usually quite innocent and quickly clear away within a week or so, they may be the first sign of some eye disorder and should always be checked with your doctor.

Q **I would like to wear contact lenses but have been told by a friend that women on the Pill often have difficulty with them.**

A The problem is that the cornea swells in response to hormone changes induced by the Pill. Hard contact lenses are more likely to give problems than the newer soft lenses. Obviously many women do wear contact lenses so you need to talk this over thoroughly with an optician who can give you proper advice.

Q **I have worn glasses since I was a child and am now in my thirties. I would like to change to contact lenses but wonder if I have left it too late.**

A Age is not the deciding factor in switching to contact lenses. Only an optician will be able to tell you if your particular prescription is suitable for contact lenses, and can explain about the various types of lenses available.

Q   **I have recently noticed thick, raised yellow patches around my eyes. They seem to be getting bigger. What are they?**

A   It sounds like xanthalasma, which is simply deposits of fatty material just under the skin. The condition itself is quite harmless but it does tend to run in families and it may be associated with high blood fat (cholesterol) levels. The only way to get rid of them is by plastic surgery, but if they are caused by high blood fat levels then they may well keep recurring unless you also change your diet.

Q   **My teenage daughter gets styes all the time. She is very upset about them so what can we do to get rid of them?**

A   A stye is simply an infection of the follicle of an eyelash. If she has frequent styes then it may be a sign that she has an infection somewhere else in her body, and it needs checking out and treating by her doctor.

Q   **What can I do for myself once I have a stye?**

A   For self help, try to prevent a stye by keeping your hands scrupulously clean and avoid touching your eyes whenever possible. Once a stye has developed you could try dissolving a teaspoon of salt in a cup of warm water and using that as an eye bath. Wrap cotton fabric round the bowl of a wooden spoon. Dip it in hot water and dab at the closed eye over the stye. This 'hot spoon' bathing is very relieving.

Q I play squash quite a lot and several players at the club have had injuries. The most common seems to be a detached retina. How would I know if this had happened to me?

A Whenever you are hit in the eye by a ball, or any object, it is important to check the injury thoroughly. Symptoms may not come on straight away, but warning signs are flashing lights, either continuously or in episodes. They may be more noticeable if you move your eyes in a particular direction. Also you may see spots before your eyes, or a sudden clouding of your vision. If you get any of these then go to your doctor, optician or hospital casualty department straight away.

Q I am a keen gardener and occasionally have scratched my eye on a twig. What is the best way of dealing with it?

A Shut your eye, pad it with fresh paper tissues, using sellotape or a plaster to keep them in place and seek immediate attention from a doctor or casualty department. Never dab at your eye with your hanky, or sleeve as you could be transferring infection into the scratch. Do not delay in seeking treatment.

Q I went recently to the doctor and he gave me antibiotic eye drops. Couldn't I have had tablets instead?

A The blood supply to the eye is so poor that antibiotics must be given directly into it. Any medicines taken by mouth will not reach the eye in high enough concentrations to be effective.

Q **What exactly is colour-blindness and how do you find out if you have it?**

A People who are affected cannot distinguish colour in the red/green spectrum. You can be tested for colour-blindness with a very simple set of cards where scattered coloured dots cover the page. A person who is not colour-blind will be able to detect certain patterns among the dots, whereas a colour-blind person will not be able to do so.

Q **Is colour-blindness hereditary?**

A Yes, it is carried by a gene that is attached to the X chromosome.

Q **Why is colour-blindness more common among men than women?**

A Women have two X chromosomes and men have one X and one Y. A woman will need two affected X chromosomes — one from her mother, the other from her father — to be colour-blind. A man needs only one affected X chromosome from either parent, and that is why this condition is very much more common in men than in women.

Ears

Q **I seem to be going a little bit deaf and I think this is due to wax in my ears. Can I get it out with some cotton buds and warm water?**

A No, and please don't attempt it. The ear canal is very narrow, so poking anything down it can only push the wax further onto the drum or cause actual tearing or even perforation. Wax must be removed by a doctor or nurse. They will syringe the ears out after the wax has been softened by drops.

Q I had an accident at work recently and received a blow over my ear. I cannot hear at all now in that ear. Will it heal?

A Any sudden increase in pressure in the ear canal can just tear the ear-drum. It normally heals on its own without any specific treatment and the hearing returns to normal, but do get this checked by your doctor.

Q What exactly is vertigo and what causes it?

A If you have vertigo it seems as if the whole room is spinning round you, or you yourself are spinning. This can cause dizziness and loss of balance and occurs because there is a disorder of the inner ear where the organs of balance are situated.

Q My ears have always stuck out and I have to wear my hair over my face so that it covers them. Is it possible to have them operated on?

A This type of surgery has excellent results once the ears are fully developed. It is a simple procedure, and because the incisions are made behind the ears no scars are visible, so you would be able to wear your hair however you wanted.

Q I went to my doctor because I'm getting a bit deaf and was told I have otosclerosis. What is this condition?

A At the entrance to the inner ear an abnormal growth of honeycombed bone occurs. This immobilizes one of the tiny bones which transmit the sound wave to the hearing nerve and you become deaf.

Q **What treatment is there for otosclerosis?**

A You will need a hearing aid at least and you may eventually need an operation.

Q **What is Meniere's Disease?**

A Sufferers complain of bouts of dizziness and hearing difficulty. These attacks can last from a few minutes to several hours, and may occur frequently or only once in a while. It is caused by an increased pressure in the labyrinth which is the organ of balance located in the inner ear.

Q **What can be done to cure Meniere's Disease?**

A In many cases it will clear up of its own accord, and if the attacks are not too drastic then lying completely still may help with the worst of the symptoms. If the vertigo is severe then drugs will be prescribed to reduce the excess fluid, and in extreme cases surgery or ultrasound can be used.

Q **I seem to have a permanent buzzing sound in my ear, almost like a wasp. What's causing it?**

A This is labelled tinnitus and there are many different causes — although in the vast majority of people who complain of tinnitus no cause is found.

Skin and hair

Our skin is a tough, waterproof and elastic outer covering which protects all our internal organs and tissues. It is an important sense organ through which we feel heat, cold, pain and touch. Hair is rooted in our skin and is supplied with blood vessels and nerve fibres which nourish the root, although the hair itself is dead. Hair is found on nearly every part of the body, except for the palms of our hands and soles of the feet.

Skin

Q **I have some patches of dry skin on my face which have proved very difficult to shift. My friend has told me that you can get hydrocortizone cream over the counter now. Do you think this would help?**

A You can buy one per cent hydrocortizone cream without a doctor's prescription. *But*, it should not be used on your face unless you have taken a doctor's advice. Facial skin is very sensitive and too much of the cream can permanently damage it.

Q **I have been shaving my legs and underarms for the past ten years or so but suddenly I have started to itch a day or so later. Why is this?**

A It is difficult to say why. If you have changed your soap or deodorant recently then you could be reacting to that. If not, then the best thing would be to stop shaving and let the hair grow. If your skin is still sensitive after a few weeks then you might try an alternative method of hair removal such as waxing.

Q I have a lot of hair on my legs which is quite dark and coarse. I used a depilatory cream, which the instructions said to leave on for five minutes. The hair hadn't really come off then so I left it for another ten. I got a nasty mark, like a burn, on one part of my leg. Do all creams do this?

A Depilatory creams, or lotions, should be used *exactly* as the instructions state. They are made from chemicals which, if your skin is sensitive, or you leave them on too long, can irritate or burn the skin. When used as directed they are perfectly safe.

Q I get confused between eczema and dermatitis. Which is which?

A They are both aspects of exactly the same condition. Dermatitis is used to describe the acute condition of swelling, redness and blistering of the skin. Eczema describes the chronic long-standing condition with ugly scratch marks and thick, dry patches of skin. Whichever you suffer from the skin itches, and it's the continuous cycle of itching and scratching that makes the condition so very miserable, as well as being unattractive to look at.

Q My eczema gets much better when I stay with my aunt who lives in an area where the water is very soft. Does this really make a difference?

A Soft water does seem to help many eczema sufferers and, if possible, it would be worth considering installing a domestic water softening scheme. Check with various manufacturers because some of them do give discounts to patients who need this facility on medical grounds.

Q My doctor says I have allergic dermatitis. I am using a new deodorant, but have had that for a few weeks, and anyway the rash is on my back. Surely I can't be allergic to this?

A Allergic dermatitis is caused by actual contact with an irritating substance such as soap, washing powder or even an allergy to a particular substance like nickel which is used in things like bra straps. Unfortunately it can take a week or longer for this form of dermatitis to develop and the skin affected isn't necessarily the part that was in contact with the allergen.

Q When I changed to a new soap I came out in a terrible rash. But how can I be certain it was the soap that caused it?

A The only way of being sure it was the soap is a process of trial and error. Do not use it for at least a fortnight and do not introduce any other new products into your routine. Then go back and use the soap and see what happens.

Q A man in my office has terrible dermatitis on his hands. I am always handling paper that he has passed to me and am worried because he doesn't seem to wash his hands all that frequently. Can I catch something from him?

A No. Eczema and dermatitis are not contagious or infectious and are not caused by any lack of personal cleanliness.

Q **I have very troublesome eczema and, although it is very well controlled, I wonder if there is something in my diet that is aggravating it?**

A Eczema is the outward visible sign of a whole variety of sensitivities, with different ones affecting different people. It could possibly be something in your diet, but you need to talk to your doctor or contact the Eczema Society.

Q **My mother-in-law has psoriasis. It looks the same as eczema to me, so what is the difference?**

A To the casual observer it can look similar, but the two conditions are quite different. In psoriasis the normal replacement that takes place in the skin all over our bodies is speeded up in certain patches. In these areas the skin appears deep pink and raised up, just as it would under a newly-healed scab. Our skin cells normally contain a lot of keratin, which makes them tough and resistant. But in psoriasis, keratin production is deficient so that all the newly-made cells in the abnormal patch of skin are very short-lived and flake off. In eczema the areas of abnormal skin are often very irritating and show signs of being scratched.

Q **My mother and her sister both have psoriasis. Does this mean it's hereditary?**

A It does tend to run in families and it seems that inherited skin types play a part in the development of this condition.

Q **I work with someone with very bad psoriasis and I am worried whether I will get it too.**

A Psoriasis is not contagious and you cannot catch it from anyone else.

Q **I have small patches of psoriasis on the front of my knees. In summer I do enjoy swimming in the sea, but am worried in case it makes the psoriasis worse.**

A There is no need to worry. Regular swimming will improve your general health and many psoriasis sufferers find seawater beneficial.

Q **Is there anything you can do to help yourself with psoriasis?**

A Sunlight seems to be good for a great many sufferers, but in the winter months it may be worth seeing if your local hospital has an artificial sunlight unit. If not it is possible to buy individual units which can be used at home.

Q I have severe eczema for which I take steroids. The doctor says I must carry a card with me, in case of an accident, which says that I take steroids regularly. Why do I need to do this?

A One of the main problems with taking steroids as a medicine is that it suppresses the natural production of the adrenal glands. When we get infections or suffer from injury our bodies have to swing into action to combat it. Much of this reaction is organized by the naturally occurring steroids made in the adrenal glands. If you are taking steroids then you are unable to do this and it is essential that in the event of an accident any emergency treatment will include a shot of steroids to help your system cope with the injury. It is for this reason that you must carry a card stating exactly what medicine and dosage you are taking.

Q I stopped taking steroids six months ago. Do I still need to carry a warning card?

A The suppressant effect of the steroids can last for several months after you have finished taking them, so you must still inform anyone giving you medical treatment if you have been on steroids in the last year.

Q I have taken steroid tablets for a skin complaint which has now cleared up. Can I just stop taking them?

A No, steroids must be withdrawn gradually. This allows your adrenal glands time to recover and start producing their own hormones.

Q **What exactly is acne?**

A Acne can occur as blackheads, whiteheads, small spots, large spots and cystic pustules. All these problems develop in the hair follicles and their associated sebaceous glands, and in the sweat glands. The normal bacteria which cover the whole of our skin invade the hair follicles and act directly on the sebum causing its breakdown into irritating chemicals which are then secreted onto the skin. These irritating chemicals are caused by a combination of bacteria and sebum together and these form the basis of all the varieties of acne.

Q **I am in my twenties but am still plagued by acne. What can I do about it?**

A Antibacterial treatments can reduce the bacterial component which is causing the acne. Your doctor may prescribe either antiseptic lotions applied directly to the skin or antibiotic tablets taken orally.

Q **My face is just covered in whiteheads. What can I do about them?**

A For this type of acne, cutting down on the production of sebum can have dramatic results. It is the sebum which causes the extensive whiteheads of some forms of acne. There is no infection, and no amount of antibiotics will help this type of acne, but cutting down on sebum production will effect a cure and this can be done by taking an anti-sebum medication prescribed by your doctor.

Q I have quite a lot of spots which my mother used to say was due to eating chocolate. I haven't eaten any for six months and I've still got spots.

A Despite popular belief, acne is not affected by anything that you eat.

Q I have had acne since I was 16 and the only time it got better was when I was pregnant. The doctor says I should have grown out of it by now, but I am getting really fed up with it.

A If your skin improved when you were pregnant then this points to a relationship between your hormone levels and the acne. It could be a form of acne called rosacea. It would help if you had some more information about how your skin reacts in certain circumstances, whether to any medicines you have been given, if you are on the Pill and whether that affected it, and how you react to sunshine. With this information you should talk to your doctor again.

Q I have very bad acne and went to the doctor who gave me some cream. It didn't work and I haven't been back. I am too embarrassed to go out looking like this, so what can I do?

A There are many different treatments for acne and you must go back to your doctor to discuss what else you could now try. If your condition is causing you to avoid going out then you need treatment for it and, if necessary, your doctor can always refer you to a specialized dermatology department.

Q **The skin around my nose got red and blotchy and then formed a blister. This has now burst and looks really ugly. What is it?**

A This sounds like impetigo and it is most common around the nose and mouth. Once the blisters have broken, then the bare sore is swarming with bacteria which can readily infect other areas of surrounding skin. You need to see a doctor to have it treated, usually with a course of antibiotics.

Q **Can I catch impetigo from other people?**

A It is very contagious and easily passed on to other people through skin contact or sharing things like towels.

Q **What should I do about a wart on my hand?**

A You may not have to do anything. It isn't necessary to treat all warts, as between 30 and 50 per cent of them will disappear by themselves.

Q **I have had a wart on my hand for quite some time now. What causes it?**

A Warts are a common affliction caused by viruses. Many separate wart viruses can be identified, and infection by one doesn't prevent you from being infected by others.

Q **Are warts contagious?**

A Warts are contagious because they are caused by a virus. They are more likely to be passed on where the environment is moist, such as a bathroom or swimming pool.

Q **What treatment is there for warts?**

A Preparations bought in the pharmacy are effective in many cases, but if further treatment is needed then quite strong chemicals are painted on the affected area until the warts have gone. If the warts are very resistant then they can be removed surgically, or frozen off, under a local anaesthetic.

Q **I have a flat wart near my groin, above the pubic hairline. It is about half an inch square and has been there for years. It is very ugly but I am too embarrassed to see my doctor about it. Is there anything I can get from the chemist to get rid of it?**

A It sounds like a benign skin lesion. The fact that it has been there, unchanged, for some years suggests that there is no malignancy. You really should visit your doctor to discuss it because s/he can arrange for it to be removed quite easily in the out-patients department.

Q **What is a verruca?**

A It is a wart that grows on the sole of the foot. Because of its position it can't grow outwards so it is pressed inwards by the regular pressure of walking, and can be very painful because of this.

Q **I have been told I have athlete's foot, but I am certainly not the sporty kind. Where did I get it from?**

A This is a common skin infection caused by a fungus, and has nothing to do with your sporting prowess, or lack of it. This particular fungus likes warm, moist places and under the toes is an ideal place for it to grow — particularly if your feet often get hot and sweaty.

Q **Can the rest of my family catch athlete's foot from me?**

A Yes, it is contagious. You need to have your own towel, flannel and bath mat and make sure they are not used by anyone else in the family.

Q **How do you get rid of athlete's foot?**

A The treatment is to use anti-fungal powder or cream. The feet must be washed and thoroughly dried at least twice a day, with clean socks or tights put on each time. A hairdryer is an excellent way of making sure that all the cracks and crevices around your toes are thoroughly dry.

Q **I have to use cream and powder to treat my athlete's foot. It is making a terrible mess of the bedclothes and I'm sure not much is staying on my foot.**

A Try wearing cotton sports socks at night. They should keep the remedial powder and cream in place, and off the sheets.

Q **What are chilblains, and do you only get them on your feet?**

A Chilblains are the result of cold damage to the skin. They occur particularly on the hands and feet, and as well as being painful they also itch.

Q **Every year I get chilblains. They are very painful, especially at night, and I wonder what I can do to avoid them?**

A It is important to keep your hands and feet warm at all times with good clothing insulation — natural fabrics like silk and wool are better insulators than synthetics. But don't wear anything that is tight because you need to have a layer of air trapped in the insulating fabric.

Q **What can I put on my chilblains to stop the discomfort and stop them coming back?**

A There are several creams on the market that will heal the skin and remove some of the discomfort, but they only treat the condition — they don't prevent it.

Q **I have recently become friendly with a woman at work who has incredibly white skin and hair. She never seems to go outdoors much at all. Does this mean she is an albino?**

A It sounds very like it. An albino is someone without any pigment in their skin at all. Their hair is white, the skin is very pale and totally pink and the eyes also have pink irises. They can never become suntanned, and can be horrendously burned if they are exposed to the sun for any length of time.

Q **Small areas on my body have begun to lose colour and are much paler than the rest of my skin. What is causing this?**

A It may be a condition called vitiligo, and the reason for this condition is not fully understood. It may be an auto-immune condition. This means that your own body is making a substance which attacks the pigment cells in your skin. Everyone, whatever their skin colour, has these pigment cells which are responsible for producing extra pigment when a fair-skinned person goes out in the sun. Vitiligo patches cannot suntan, and in fact the skin is very sun-sensitive.

Q **I have some areas of vitiligo on my body. Will they go away eventually?**

A Although the condition can remain static, it rarely goes away once it has appeared.

Q **Is it true that sunbathing can be a possible cause of skin cancer?**

A Yes, although for anyone who spends just two weeks in the sun and otherwise gets their sun in the northern hemisphere, the risk is small.

Q **Who is most at risk from skin cancer?**

A Fair-skinned people who spend a great deal of time in the sun have the greatest risk. It is never wise to expose white skin to extreme sun (real, or artificial) in anything other than small, controlled doses.

Q What is a melanoma?

A It's the term for new, usually deeply pigmented areas on the skin — similar to moles — which can increase in size and have a raised surface. These are called melanomas.

Q Are melanomas always black?

A No, a very tiny group are not pigmented at all so any new blemish which grows, or bleeds, should be referred to your doctor.

Q I am worried about getting skin cancer. What are the early signs?

A First look for any melanomas on your skin. If the pigment is irregularly distributed, giving the spot a geographical appearance like the contour map of an island, then the spot may be malignant. One of the first changes that can happen in an already established mole is that it loses its near regular shape and colour and begins to spread around the outer edges. Such a spot may or may not bleed or crust over.

Q I have a mole that seems to be getting bigger. Should I see my doctor about it?

A If you notice any sore which fails to heal, or a mole that seems to be growing, then you should consult a doctor for a proper diagnosis as soon as possible.

Q **I have what the doctor calls a 'rodent ulcer' on my face. Can it be cured?**

A It is a form of skin cancer — also known as basal cell cancer — and is a very treatable and usually totally curable condition. It is more common in fair-skinned people who have spent a lot of time in the sunlight. Treatment is simple (usually radiotherapy) and very effective. In well over 90 per cent of cases the cancer can be totally cleared without leaving any disfiguring scars.

Q **Now I am in my sixties I have a number of large flat freckles on my hands. Are they dangerous, and will they go away?**

A These are 'sunspots' and appear on the hands and face of many people as they get older. They are not harmful but, unfortunately, they rarely go away.

Q **I seem to get a discharge from my navel. What is this?**

A Some people do have very deep and hidden navels and this can lead to the problem of skin oils and talcum powder collecting in them. It can then get infected and cause a slight discharge.

Q **How do I avoid getting a discharge from my navel?**

A After each bath you should thoroughly dry your navel and then clean it out using cotton buds and surgical spirit, or surgical spirit mixed with hititane. You can get these lotions from a pharmacist. Clean your navel gently, but firmly, and if there are any hard pieces tucked away in the crevices of your skin then ease them out gently with tweezers.

Q **What causes bedsores?**

A Bedsores occur at the contact points between body and bed — usually the buttocks, elbows and heels. The weight of the body stops the flow of blood through the tissues and the starved cells die and slough away, leaving an ulcer. These ulcers may then get infected and spread.

Q **My grandmother has recently had a stroke and will be confined to bed for several weeks. How do we prevent her getting bedsores?**

A Simple approaches to preventing bedsores are very effective, but they are time consuming. Just rub the pressure spots briskly for five to ten minutes every one or two hours. To rub the patient's bottom, first lie her on one side and then the other. In this way both the hips and spine can be completely massaged without disturbing the patient too much.

Q **My mother has been confined to bed for some time. She does get very hot and sweaty and the nurse said she will need extra care to avoid bedsores. What can I do to help her?**

A Bedsores are made worse if the skin is soggy with sweat, so massage with alcohol or surgical spirit and dry off the area with a non-perfumed talcum powder. A real sheepskin next to the skin will keep it dry and prevent pressure.

Q **Every year I get one or two crops of cold sores round my mouth. Why do I keep getting them?**

A Cold sores are caused by one of the herpes viruses and once they are in your system you can never quite get rid of them.

Q **Can people catch cold sores from me?**

A The sores are very infectious during their weeping and blistering stage so don't kiss anyone, particularly babies, and be very careful to keep your face flannel, towel, and handkerchiefs exclusively for your own use.

Q **What's the best way of treating cold sores?**

A You can get a wide range of creams, lotions and ointments from the pharmacist that will dry up your cold sores and ease the pain. If the cold sores are very persistent, consult your doctor because you may need an anti-viral drug to clear them up.

Q **I very rarely get a cold, but I still get cold sores. Why is this?**

A Although these sores are usually triggered by a simple cold virus, hence the name, they can also be brought on by things like intense sunlight or extreme cold.

Q **I never used to get cold sores at all, but since I have been on a strict diet I seem to get quite a few.**

A Cold sores can be associated with certain vitamin deficiencies. Check that your diet is not so strict that you are not getting the essential nutrients that your body needs. Try to aim for a good balanced diet, high in fresh fruit and vegetables.

Q **Is there a natural remedy for cold sores?**

A You could try Tea Tree oil. If you apply it externally to the sores every hour it will help reduce the pain and accelerate the healing. Lavender water used in the same way is also effective.

Q **Every winter my lips get very cracked and dry, especially if I have a cold. Can I do anything to prevent this?**

A Not really, winter is a hard time for your skin because the cold weather and winds dry out your skin very quickly. Applying lip salve or petroleum jelly regularly may give you some protection and ease the soreness.

Q **I get very fed up when I have a cold because my nose goes bright red. What can I do about it?**

A It depends on how heavy your cold is. If the skin is broken and sore because you are blowing your nose a lot, then really you should not put anything on your skin at all. If it is just red, then a green colour corrective cream worn under your usual foundation should do the trick.

Q **Why are my shoes always tight in hot weather? Sometimes it is so bad that I get blisters.**

A Feet tend to swell in hot weather and you should allow for this when buying shoes. Before you do any walking in new shoes try to wear them around the house first, to see where any sore spots are likely to be. You can then catch it before it blisters and put on a protective plaster to cushion it.

Q **I seem to get a lot of blisters on my heels in the summer. Some get quite big and I wonder if I should burst them?**

A It is not a good idea to burst a blister unless absolutely necessary, as it increases the risk of infection.

Q **I had a terrible blister when on a walking holiday last year. I had to burst it, it was so bad, but what is the proper procedure in case I ever have to do it again?**

A If it is really essential that you burst a blister, then sterilize a large needle by boiling it or passing it through a flame until it is red hot. When it has cooled down, clean the area with antiseptic lotion and then pierce the blister twice and wipe away the fluid on cotton wool or clean tissue. Cover the area immediately with a sterile, dry dressing and keep it covered until it has healed.

Q **What immediate treatment should you give for a burn?**

A The instant treatment of a minor burn or scald is to cool the area and stop the heat damage spreading within the skin. Immediately plunge the burned or scalded part into cold water and if possible add ice to this water. Running tap water is colder than static water.

Q **What sort of dressing should I put on a scald or burn?**

A Once the area is thoroughly cooled (see previous question), allow the skin to dry in the open air. If there is blistering, or the skin is broken, cover with a simple cotton dressing; do not use lint or cotton wool as this will stick and be uncomfortable to remove.

Q My grandmother always says you should put butter on burns. Is that the right thing to do?

A You should not put butter or any ointments, creams or lotions on a burn. If possible, cool the skin at once with ice or running cold water.

Q My mother was badly burned in the kitchen when some oil in a pan caught fire. What could I have done to help her?

A The first thing to do is cover the burning pan with a lid, or some other cover. Never put it under a tap — the water will immediately become steam and spread the fire all over the room. The next most important thing is to get the patient away from the source of damage as quickly as possible. Smother all burning clothes at once to completely deprive the fire of air. See the previous questions for how to deal with a burn.

Q Is it all right to give painkillers to someone who has been burned?

A It may help to give painkillers so that any subsequent dressings will be less uncomfortable. These can be repeated every four hours.

Q Is it always necessary to go to hospital for treatment for a burn?

A If the burned area is large, or the burn is deep with clothing stuck to it, then it must be treated in hospital.

Q If someone is burned should you try to get their clothes off or leave them as they are?

A Never attempt to peel off burnt, stuck-on clothing as you will probably peel off areas of damaged skin as well.

Q My husband sometimes bites me when we are making love. It's not deep, but it does break the skin and when my sister saw it she said I should have antibiotics. Surely that is not necessary?

A The mouth is a rich source of bacteria. Saliva is made up of normal body fluids and contains any infections — virus or bacteria — which are present in the rest of the body and around the gums and teeth. Given these facts, it is a general rule of thumb that all human bites should be given antibiotics.

Q I have just bought a kitten and she tends to bite and scratch quite a lot. Do I need antibiotics for these bites?

A Animal bites are much less likely to get infected as a general rule, so you probably just need to give it a good clean with an antiseptic lotion.

Q I have an ulcer on my leg that doesn't seem to be healing all that well. Why is it taking so long?

A Leg ulcers can be very difficult to heal. Poor nutrition can play a part and infection can be a major reason for delayed healing. The most important factor of all is a poor blood supply to the affected area.

Q **What can I do to help my leg ulcer to heal?**

A It is important to keep the ulcer at a constant temperature and not allow the area to get cold, or too hot. It is also important to raise the leg off the ground whenever you can, on a footstool or sofa, but this doesn't mean never getting any exercise. In fact regular exercise for ten minutes an hour will increase the pulse rate of the whole body, thus increasing the blood flow through the skin and muscles of the leg. This will then aid the healing process. New seaweed dressings are proving very effective for long-standing ulcers.

Q **Is it all right to use a hot water bottle next to my leg, to help the ulcer to heal?**

A Hot water bottles and electric fires can damage the new growing skin around an ulcer and should be avoided at all costs.

Q **How do you avoid getting ingrowing toenails?**

A They usually only affect the big toe and are caused when the edge of the nail digs deeply into the quick at the side and causes an infection. Careful cutting of the nails, making sure not to prod or poke the quick, and cutting the toenail straight across instead of in a curved fashion, will usually be enough to avoid this problem.

Q **What is a whitlow?**

A It is when the quick around the nail is infected. The medical term is paronychia — 'para' means beside and 'onychia' is the nail.

Q I would like to know what the treatment is for a whitlow.

A If the infection comes to a head it may have to be lanced, because if left untreated it can lead to an infection which spreads through the body.

Q I have noticed that my nails have become very pitted and scarred recently. What could be causing it?

A It could be an infection caused by a fungus, the same one that causes athlete's foot. The nail may also become very uncomfortable.

Q What is the treatment for pitted nails?

A Treatment is with anti-fungal powders and creams, but the condition won't disappear overnight as it can take several months for the damaged nail to grow out.

Q My fingernails are quite brittle and break easily. How can I get them to grow?

A First check that you are eating the right things to encourage your nails. For growth you need a balanced diet, high in the vitamins and minerals that come from eating protein, fruit and vegetables. Calcium is essential, as is Vitamin A which helps prevent nails splitting. Iodine, found in kelp, also promotes growth.

Q I wear nail polish on my fingers and toes all the time but my mother says it will damage them. Is she right?

A The nail polish itself will not cause you any harm, but it is not a good idea to have the whole nail area covered all the time. A chance for the air to get at the nail, and nail bed, is essential to keep the nails healthy.

Hair

Q Since I started taking drugs recently prescribed by my doctor I notice that I have grown more facial hair. My doctor has said it is not important, but is there anything I can do about it?

A It is difficult to say without knowing exactly what drugs you are taking. Some hormone replacement therapies and steroid treatments can sometimes increase activity of the hair follicle and stimulate more hair growth. If the hair is distressing to you, then it is important. Go back to your doctor and ask if your drugs contain any of the steroids or hormones that might be causing this. Then see whether there is any alternative treatment available to you.

Q I have got very bad dandruff. Is it caused by using too strong a shampoo?

A Dandruff is excessive flaking of the skin on the scalp, so unless you happen to be allergic to one of the components in the shampoo you are using there is no way that it can cause, or increase your dandruff. The important thing is that you always rinse your hair thoroughly.

Q **What is the best way to get rid of dandruff?**

A Use any good dandruff shampoo, as directed, and wash your hair every two or three days. Make sure you rinse the shampoo out thoroughly, using only clean water — so do not wash your hair in the bath. For a week or two you should avoid using things like mousse or gel on your hair, as you may be allergic to the perfume in some of these products. It would be sensible to avoid them until your dandruff has cleared up.

Q **Is it possible for women to go bald?**

A Hair loss is not uncommon in women. It may be related to an actual disease such as thyroid deficiency, some severe anaemias, or fungal infections of the scalp, or it may happen for no apparent reason at all.

Q **I am only 23, but my hair is coming out in handfuls and I have no idea why. What can I do?**

A First, do go and see your doctor. Take with you a day's collection of hair if you think that your hair loss is not obvious enough. There are very few treatable conditions which cause sudden hair loss. Thyroid disease and severe blood loss might just possibly cause it, but these conditions would be fairly obvious to you, even if you're not a doctor. Or you may be developing alopecia, a very unpredictable condition which we know little about and can treat even less. So there are just no easy answers for this distressing condition.

Q **I have recently developed a large bald patch on my head. I thought this only happened to men. Will it eventually go away?**

A This condition is called alopecia areata and women are more likely to suffer from it than men. The hair usually regrows after many months, but then a new patch often occurs. Unfortunately there is no easy treatment to overcome the problem. It has been suggested that it is an auto-immune disease and that this affects the hair follicles and prevents growth.

Q **My daughter is having treatment for cancer. Part of the treatment involves chemicals which, we have been told, may make her hair fall out. She seems more devastated by this than anything else. Is there anything that can be done to prevent it happening?**

A A Cold Cap can be very effective in preventing hair loss in these circumstances. Just before treatment she must thoroughly wet her hair and put ear muffs on to protect her ears. Then next to her scalp is placed either a commercially available Cold Cap or ice cubes in a plastic bag. This is left in place during treatment and for 30 to 50 minutes afterwards.

Q **How does keeping the scalp cold help in preventing hair loss when undergoing radiotherapy?**

A By reducing the blood supply to the scalp. This means that less of the harmful chemicals will reach the hair follicle and damage it.

Brain and nervous system

A healthy nervous system is truly the foundation of good health. It is through our nervous system that we adapt ourselves to our environment and to all external stimuli. It is when we are not functioning well that everyday stresses become magnified and we can have problems in dealing with our everyday life.

Sleep

Q **I am not sleeping as much as I used to when I was younger. Is this normal?**

A Sleep patterns do change with age and the amount of physical and mental exercise you get during the day. As we get older we do need less sleep and if you have a lifestyle that offers little or no physical or mental exertion then you are more likely to cat-nap during the day and thus have poor sleep at night.

Q **I know we have different types of sleep, but what exactly are they?**

A Sleep can be described as a series of peaks and troughs in our consciousness level. There are times when we are in shallow sleep and this is when a noise will waken us. Also our eyes move rapidly underneath the closed lids, so this is called Rapid Eye Movement (REM) sleep. If you are woken during this type of sleep you wake easily and can recall what you were dreaming about. Deep sleep occurs between episodes of REM and is usually at its deepest within an hour or two of going to sleep. If you are woken then you will be groggy and thick-headed, unable to remember what you were dreaming and not functioning very accurately for a while.

Q I sleep for eight hours a night but I read about politicians and similar people who only get four to six hours. Surely it must affect their health?

A Our patterns of sleep develop during childhood and we all have different expectations. Adequate amounts of sleep are certainly essential for healthy living, but anything between four and ten hours a night is entirely 'normal', provided that this is what the individual requires.

Q I spend all day running around after the family and by the time I get to bed my mind is buzzing and I can't sleep. I have a cup of tea and a cigarette to calm me down, but it doesn't seem to help. Would the odd sleeping pill do the trick?

A The nicotine from the cigarette and the caffeine in your tea are both stimulants and certainly won't help you to get to sleep. It is never a good idea to take sleeping tablets regularly for this kind of wakefulness. Try a hot bath with some relaxing bath oil and a cup of camomile tea to unwind. Listen to some calming music, think of a peaceful and quiet scene and see if that helps you to drift off naturally. Or try reading a comforting, non-demanding book.

Q **I go through periods when I just don't sleep at all. Would sleeping pills be a good idea?**

A Most people have times in their lives when they can't sleep. About one in ten will suffer and for the vast majority it can be simply and effectively managed without resorting to medication. Sleeping pills are never the answer to long-term insomnia, but there is no law that says you have to lie in bed tossing and turning, get up and make a drink, read a book or watch television. It might put you to sleep faster than just lying there worrying about it.

Ailments and illness

Q **What exactly is a headache?**

A Our brain is enclosed almost totally in a bony shell — the skull — to protect this vital organ. Any alteration in the tension or pressure within the skull is reflected in changes in the brain cells. Low pressure, or high pressure, can both give problems and are responsible for many headaches.

Q **Are all headaches the same?**

A There are several types of headache: the headache associated with a hangover comes from a combination of dehydration and the toxins in the alcohol; headaches brought on by hormonal changes around the time of menstruation can sometimes be alleviated by taking the oral contraceptive, but then again in some women sensitivity to progesterone itself can bring on a headache; dietary allergies can frequently bring on headaches, cheese, caffeine and red wine are common culprits.

Q **I have always been a fairly tense sort of person and recently I have been getting a lot of headaches. Is this due to my tension?**

A It might be, or it might not. If you start getting headaches when you have not had any before, then you must have them checked out by your doctor. There are many causes of headaches and you need to exclude the more serious ones before you label them as just tension.

Q **When I have a headache I frequently feel sick as well, so taking painkillers is a waste of time because I just vomit them up again. Is there anything else I can try?**

A Using soluble brands of analgesic helps; and many proprietary preparations are mixed with an anti-emetic which also aids absorption. The best solution is an analgesic rectal suppository. The drug is quickly absorbed into the system, but there are no ill effects for the stomach. In mainland Europe they are the normal preparation for this kind of problem so you could try asking your pharmacist if he can get hold of some for you. Failing that, if you take a holiday abroad you could buy some there.

Q **I often have splitting headaches and take quite a few painkillers to get them under control. My flatmate says that I shouldn't just go on taking tablets for it.**

A She's right that you shouldn't be putting up with regular headaches. You should see your doctor and have a thorough check-up. It is always a bad idea to take any painkiller regularly unless it has been prescribed by your doctor.

Q I often take paracetamol at work if I get a headache, but my boss has told me they can be dangerous if I take a lot of them. Is this true?

A Paracetamol can certainly be very dangerous if taken in quantities large enough to cause an overdose. Irreversible kidney damage and even death can occur some days after an apparently full recovery.

Q I work with a girl who suffers from migraine several times a month. What exactly is wrong with her?

A The term migraine is much misused and has come to mean anything from a severe headache to a full-blown migraine. Many severe attacks of migraine are heralded by disturbances of vision such as flashing lights, or seeing things in a distorted way. The headaches are usually on one side of the head and can be accompanied by nausea and vomiting.

Q I have heard that cheese or chocolate can trigger off a migraine attack, is this true?

A It is not the only factor, but something in your diet can precipitate a migraine. It is often related to an allergy to a food or substance, and the sufferer has to experiment to find out just what causes an attack and then avoid it.

Q I have always been a fairly anxious sort of person, but as I have settled down and had a family it seems to have got worse. Should I see a doctor?

A Everyone is anxious at some point in their lives, but the first thing to do is to identify the real cause of the problem and, if possible, remove it. If your worries are connected with your family then try to confide in someone and talk them through. Learning to relax is also important and you could try a number of different techniques like yoga, meditation or an aromatherapy massage. See which works for you, and certainly talk to your doctor about it, but unless your anxiety is acute it is worth trying to cope without drugs if you can. Many drugs used to treat anxiety become less effective with continued use and the dose may need to be increased. Also some of these drugs have side-effects which can cause anxiety symptoms themselves when you stop taking them.

Q People talk a lot about being 'depressed', but what exactly are the symptoms?

A Depression is a strange disease and has many forms. It can range in severity from very mild disturbance to deep depression and intense anxiety. The classical early signs are sleeplessness, early waking, bodily sluggishness — usually showing itself as constipation, a diminished sex drive, reduced accuracy in everyday performance and the inability to make simple everyday decisions.

Q **The doctor has arranged for me to have a CAT scan and I am not sure just what is involved.**

A CAT stands for Computerized Axial Tomography and is a major improvement on the techniques available for studying soft tissues like the brain. It uses X-ray beams to construct a continuous picture of any part of your body. When having a CAT scan you lie perfectly still on a table while a large arc, containing the X-ray beam, passes over you. It can take up to 20 minutes but the machine never actually touches you and there is absolutely no discomfort involved.

Q **My mother recently had what I thought was a stroke, but the doctor called a transient ischaemic attack. What exactly did she have?**

A A transient ischaemic attack is a warning which may herald the likelihood that the sufferer will get a 'real' stroke later on. There is usually paralysis or other difficulty and it does appear exactly like a stroke, but there is complete recovery within 24 hours.

Q **I had a mild stroke earlier this year and although I am making a good recovery I would like to know exactly what caused it.**

A Basically, a stroke is the result of damage to part of the brain caused by an interruption to its blood supply. This can be caused by a clot (cerebral thrombosis or infarction) or by possible bleeding (cerebral haemorrhage). Only very rarely does it happen as a result of injury. There are so many causes of a stroke that it may not be possible to pinpoint the exact problem.

Q A number of people in my family have had strokes and they have all been affected in different ways. Is there no common factor?

A A stroke can affect movement or sensation in any part of the body. It can affect any one of the senses as well as memory, emotions or even thinking. Any one, or a number, of these effects may be apparent in the sufferer and the combinations can be endless.

Q Are strokes always fatal?

A No, by no means, but the outcome is not always predictable. In some severe cases the patient does not regain consciousness and dies within a day or two. In other cases there can be a marked improvement in condition as the healthy parts of the brain learn to take over some of the functions of the damaged area, so that the patient makes a complete recovery. Between these extremes every permutation is possible.

Q Is there a 'type' of person who is more likely to have a stroke?

A They are more common in overweight, under-exercised elderly smokers. Raised blood pressure can also be a contributory factor.

Q What is epilepsy?

A There are many different degrees of epilepsy and a large number of causes. The seizure itself is due to an abnormal discharge of impulses from some part of the brain. The extent and site of this abnormal area determines the quality of the seizure.

Q **What happens during an epileptic attack?**

A If it is a major attack, or *grand mal* as it is known, then it will involve loss of consciousness together with spasmodic muscle contractions and sometimes loss of control of the bladder. In a minor attack, or *petit mal*, there may be only a very slight 'absence' for perhaps just a second or two. About two in every five epileptic fits occur during sleep when the brain is switched off from any obvious activity.

Q **What treatment is there for epilepsy?**

A Firstly there needs to be a thorough search for the cause of the epilepsy. If no such cause is discovered then anticonvulsants and sedatives are usually prescribed. They act on the brain to stop the abnormal nervous activity. The amount of medicine needed will vary enormously, both with the frequency and severity of the problem, and with the tolerance and body weight of the sufferer.

Q **I work with a woman who has multiple sclerosis. I am not sure exactly what the disease is and I do not like to ask her directly.**

A Multiple sclerosis, or MS, is an unpredictable and sometimes fatal disease. Sufferers develop plaques of sclerosed tissue on and within the insulation (myelin) sheaths of the nerve fibres. These plaques interfere with the transmission of impulses along the nerves. This has the effect of giving odd sensations, or preventing certain muscles from functioning.

Q **What is the usual progress of MS?**

A It is a very variable disease both in the extent of the damage it does to any particular individual and the way in which it progresses. There are periods of spontaneous remission, from a few months to several years, when the symptoms may disappear entirely. There are also people who have only one episode of the disease and do not progress to develop full-blown MS. About one-third of known MS sufferers can work for 15 years or more after their diagnosis.

Q **How can I be tested to see if I have MS?**

A There is no simple test that can check whether a person has MS or not, since although CAT scanning is very accurate at showing where plaque exists, it is only applicable to people who have symptoms suggestive of MS.

Q **I was recently diagnosed as suffering from MS, but my doctor has not offered me any treatment. Is there anything I can do for myself?**

A With a disease where there is no general recognized treatment it can be hard for doctors to suggest how you should manage your illness. It is a good idea to find out as much about it as possible through reading, and contacting other sufferers.

Q My granddaughter is 22 years old and has just been diagnosed as suffering from schizophrenia. This is an illness we know nothing about, but we would like to be of some practical help to her. What can we do?

A Schizophrenia is a very puzzling and disabling mental illness. There are about 250,000 sufferers in Britain and at any one time around 20,000 are receiving hospital treatment. The schizophrenic becomes quite divorced from reality. Her actions and mental processes just do not balance with the situation as the rest of us see it. This dissociation is what makes the problem so very difficult for the sufferer's friends and relatives. Try to find a local support group and ask for their help.

Q My sister has a history of mental illness. Recently she became very ill and, against her will, was taken into hospital. Can you be taken in without your permission?

A Yes, under very special circumstances, patients can be taken into psychiatric care even if they don't want to go. In the UK, the conditions are laid down very strictly by the Mental Health Act, and the most common reason is if a doctor believes the patient is a danger to themselves or to others. If you have any worries about your sister being detained, ask to speak to the sister or the psychiatric social worker on the ward, or contact MIND.

Q What is Alzheimer's disease?

A This name used to be given to pre-senile dementia. That is dementia which comes on in middle age, rather than in the elderly. It is now quite widely used to describe any dementia in adults which has no obvious cause.

Q **My mother is only 49, but has Alzheimer's Disease. Does it usually hit people so young?**

A Alzheimer's Disease is just one of several conditions which can lead to the impairment of brain function and, although it is rare, it can occur in people from 40 upwards.

Q **My mother, who is 75, has become very forgetful and confused recently. Is this the beginning of senile dementia?**

A Those are certainly some of the symptoms of senile dementia, along with disorientation and being unable to carry out simple tasks. With this disease the brain has ceased to function appropriately, but there are many reversible causes of dementia and these should all be explored first. Potential thyroid disorder, acute infection, heart failure, strokes and some medicines can all give symptoms which mimic dementia. With elderly people it can also be hard to separate 'true' dementia from simple depression, so it is important to see your doctor and get a proper diagnosis.

Q **My mother has just developed Parkinson's disease, and although she is not badly affected at the moment I am very worried that I may catch it. I am now aged 55 and responsible for the care of my mother, so obviously I cannot afford to be ill myself.**

A Parkinson's disease is a very variable condition, but it is in no way contagious and cannot be passed from one person to another.

Q **I find Parkinson's disease rather frightening. What causes it?**

A The condition is due to the gradual deterioration of the nerve control of some muscles. This means that the nerve impulses, which control the contraction and relaxation of muscles, are delayed or misplaced. Muscles contract for too long and then relax too suddenly so that instead of the normal smooth action, movements are jerky and somewhat uncontrolled. There are also a lot of involuntary movements such as tremor of the head and hands.

Q **I have just been diagnosed as having Parkinson's disease and am concerned about how quickly my condition will deteriorate.**

A The disease starts very slowly indeed, and it may be several years before a minor problem progresses to the stage where the illness is very difficult to cope with. There are many useful medicines which will control the disease for a long time.

Q **Can I do anything to help my mother who is in the early stages of Parkinson's disease?**

A The most important thing is to encourage her to carry on with as much normal day-to-day occupation as possible. She must continue to go out walking, or even better, take up swimming. Keeping all the joints flexible and mobile is very important. In the later stages of the illness, the loss of muscle control can make walking difficult because sufferers seem unable to get their centre of gravity in the right place and are very unsteady on their feet. So your mother should use a stick as a steadying agent, inside and outside the house. Obviously, your mother will be on medicines to help her condition and you should ensure that she takes them regularly.

Dependency

Q I have been taking sleeping pills for three years since my husband died. I realize that I shouldn't need them any more, but how do I give them up?

A It is very natural to take sleeping pills at that crucial time in your life, but by doing so you have not returned to your own natural sleep pattern. The best way to do this is to start by cutting down the tablets very slowly. If you can, break a tablet into halves and quarters and for the first two weeks take only three-quarters of a tablet. Then cut back to only half a tablet for the next few weeks, and when you are comfortable cut down to a quarter. Keep at this reduced rate for a while, then only take it every other night until you feel able to stop altogether.

Q I have been taking tranquillizers prescribed by my doctor for a number of years. I am worried about being on them for so long, so is it all right if I stop taking them?

A Stopping tranquillizers can be a real problem. It is very important not to stop suddenly because the side-effects of a sudden withdrawal can be alarming and even result in major convulsions which can be life-threatening. It is important to reduce your dosage in a planned, ordered way and this must be discussed with your doctor. The time it will take you to stop taking tranquillizers depends very much on the dose you are taking at present. Generally, the larger the dose the longer the time needed to stop.

Q **Is there any assistance available to help people who are coming off tranquillizers?**

A Self-help groups can be a great support in this situation. Talk to your doctor and see if s/he knows of any local groups.

Q **My sister and her husband are both alcoholics. They don't want to discuss it, or get any help. Is there anything the family can do?**

A It is an uphill task to give up alcohol. Recognizing that you have a problem is an essential first step in that process. There are agencies that can help them, if they want that, but if you give them both all the support you can, while making it clear that you do not condone their drinking, then that is probably as much as you can do. It is also a mistake to prop them up and protect them from the results of their alcoholism. This may be a 'kind' reaction, but you are only delaying the time when they must face up to their addiction.

Q **I like to have a drink after work with my colleagues, but I seem to be drinking more than usual. How much is it safe to drink?**

A Alcohol is a brain depressant which slowly but surely suppresses our abilities and skills. It is one of the commonest drugs of abuse in our society. How 'safe' it is depends a lot on your own body tolerance for alcohol and exactly how much you are drinking. It is usually recognized that for women two and a half units of alcohol a day on a regular basis is too much. A unit is half a pint of beer or a single spirit. The other way to see how dependent you are on alcohol is to go for seven clear days without any — if you can't do this then you do have a problem and should seek help.

Information register

Whatever health problem you may have, there is usually a support group or information centre available to give advice and help. Your own doctor, hospital, or even local library, will often be able to give you a list of people who may be able to assist you or put you in touch with those who also share your concern. Many of the organizations or individuals in this listing are charities working on a very restricted budget. It would help them if you would enclose an SAE when writing.

Useful addresses in the UK

General health

Arthritis Care
6 Grosvenor Crescent, London SW1X 7ER (071 235 0902)
Arthritis and Rheumatism Council
41 Eagle St, London WC1 4AR (071 405 8572)
Asthma Society
300 Upper St, London N1 2XX (071 226 2260)
Asthma Swim Movement
45 Lickhill Road, Calne, Wilts SN11 9EZ
Autistic Society
276 Willesden Lane, London NW2 5RB (081 451 3844)
Back Pain Association
31-33 Park Road, Teddington, Middlesex TW11 0AB (081 977 5474)
Charcot Marie Tooth Disease Society
c/o Ivor Dartnall-Smith, 73 Watson Close, Upavon, Pewsey, Wilts SN9 6AF
Chest, Heart and Stroke Association
Tavistock House North, Tavistock Square, London WC1H 9JE (071 387 3012)
Coeliac Society
PO Box 220, High Wycombe, Bucks HP11 2HY (0494 437278)

Colitis and Crohn's Disease Association
981 London Rd, St Albans, Herts AL1 1NX
Colostomy Welfare Group
38-39 Eccleston Square, London SW1V 1PB
Cystic Fibrosis Research Trust
Alexander House, 5 Blyth Road, Bromley, Kent BR1 3RS
Diabetic Association
10 Queen Anne St, London W1M 0BD
DIALs (Disablement Information and Advice Lines)
117 High St, Clay Cross, Derbyshire S45 9DZ (0246 864498)
Disfigurement Guidance Centre
52 Crossgate, Cupar, Fife KY15 5HS (0334 55746)
Down's Syndrome Association
12/13 Clapham Common Southside, London SW4 7AA (071 720 0008)
Dyslexia Foundation
133 Gresham Rd, Staines, Middlesex TW18 2AJ (0784 59498)
Dystonia Society
Unit 32, Omnibus Workspace, 39-41 North Road, London N7 9DP
Eczema Society
Tavistock House East, Tavistock Square, London WC1H 9SR
Epilepsy Association
Anstey House, 40 Hanover Square, Leeds LS3 1BE
Foundation for the Study of Infant Deaths
15 Belgrave Square, London SW1X 8PS (071 235 1721)
Gluten Allergy information from The Coeliac Society
PO Box 220, High Wycombe, Bucks HP11 2HY (0494 437278)
Haemophilia Society
123 Westminster Bridge Road, London SE1 7HR (071 928 2020)
Healthline
18 Victoria Square, London E2 9PF (081 980 4848 — call from 2-10pm
for a full list of their information services)
Ileostomy Society
Amblehurst House, Chobham, Woking, Surrey, GU24 8PZ
Medical Advisory Service
10 Barley Mow Passage, London W4 4PH (081 994 9874)
Multiple Sclerosis Society
25 Effie Rd, London SW6 1EE (071 736 6267)
Psoriasis Association
7 Milton St, Northampton NN2 7JG (0604 711129)
Raynaud's Association Trust
40 Bladon Crescent, Alsager, Cheshire ST7 2BG (09363 5167)
Retinitis Pigmentosa Society
(0327 53276 Helpline)
Scoliosis Association
380-384 Harrow Road, London W9 2HU (071 289 5652)
Spina Bifida and Hydrocephalus Association
22 Upper Woburn Place, London WC1H 0EP (071 388 1382)
Spinal Injuries Association
76 St James's Lane, London N10 3DF (081 444 2121)
Thalassaemia Society
107 Nightingale Lane, London N8 7QY (081 348 0437)

Sexual health

Cystitis
75 Mortimer Road, London N1 5AR (071 249 8664)
Endometriosis Society
65 Holmdene Avenue, Herne Hill, London SE24 9LD (071 737 4764)
Family Planning Information Service
27-35 Mortimer St, London W1N 7RJ (071 636 7866)
Foresight Association for Preconceptual Care
The Old Vicarage, Church Lane, Witley, Godalming, Surrey GU8 5PN
Hysterectomy Support Group
11 Henryson Rd, Brockley, London SE4 1HL
National Childbirth Trust
9 Queensborough Terrace, London W2 3TB (071 221 3833)
Natural Family Planning Association
28 Dooley Drive, Old Rd, Merseyside, L30 8RS (051 526 7663)
Pregnancy Advisory Service
11-13 Charlotte St, London W1P 1ND (071 637 8962)
Premenstrual Syndrome National Association
2nd Floor, 25 Market St, Guildford, Surrey GU1 4LB (0483 572715)
Stillbirth and Neonatal Deaths Society
28 Portland Place, London W1N 3DE (071 436 5881)
Terrence Higgins Trust
BM AIDS, London WC1N 3XX (071 242 1010 Helpline)
Women's Health Concern
17 Earls Terrace, London W8 6LP (071 602 6669)

Cancer

BACUP (British Association of Cancer United Patients)
121/123 Charterhouse St, London EC1M 6AA (071 608 1661)
Breast Care and Mastectomy Association (BCMA)
26a Harrison Street, Kings Cross, London WC1H 8JG (071 837 0908)
Cancer Link
17 Britannia St, London WC1X 9JN (071 833 2451)
Women's National Cancer Control Campaign
Telephone helpline available 9.30-4.30 weekdays (071 495 4995)

Addiction/dependency/mental illness

Accept Drugs Helpline
470 Harrow Road, London W9 (071 286 3339)
Al-Anon Family Groups and Alateen
61 Great Dover St, London SE1 4YF (071 403 0888)
Alcohol Concern
305 Gray's Inn Road, London WC1X 8QF (071 833 3471)
Alcoholics Anonymous
PO Box 1, 11 Redcliffe Gardens, London SW10 9BQ (071 352 3001)
Alzheimer's Disease Society
3rd Floor, Bank Buildings, Fulham Broadway, London SW6 1EP (071 381 3177)

Anorexic Family Aid Information Centre
44-48 Magdalen St, Norwich NR3 1JE (0603 621414)
ASH (Action on Smoking and Help)
5-11 Mortimer Street, London W1N 7RH (071 637 9843)
DAWN (Drugs, Alcohol Women, Nationally)
Omnibus Workspace, 39-41 North Road, London N7 9DP (071 700 4653)
Mental Health Foundation
8 Hallan St, London W1N 6DH (071 580 0145)
MIND (the National Association for Mental Health)
22 Harley St, London W1N 2ED (071 637 0741)
Schizophrenia Fellowship
78 Victoria Road, Surbiton, Surrey KT6 4NS (081 390 3651)
TRANX (Self-help groups for those with tranquillizer addiction)
17 Peel Road, Wealdstone, Harrow HA3 7QX (071 427 2065)

Useful addresses in Australia

General health

Allergy Association
PO Box 298, Ringwood, Victoria 3134 (03 720 3215)
Arthritis Foundation
2 Angel Place, Sydney 2000 (221 2456)
Association of Self-help Groups
39 Dargham Street, Glebe 2037 (660 6136)
Asthma Foundation
1 Angel Place, Sydney 2000 (235 1293)
Coeliac Society
10 Diana Avenue, West Pymble 2073 (498 2593)
Colostomy Association
630 George St, Sydney 2000 (264 2741)
Multiple Sclerosis Society
5 Bryson St, Chatswood 2067 (412 1577)
National Heart Foundation
343 Riley St, Surrey Hills 2010 (211 5188)
Stroke Recovery Association
1 Bedford St, Surrey Hills 2010 (699 4096)

Sexual health

Abortion Access, Advice Care Centre and Referral
PO Box 116, Woollahra 2025 (484 7455)
Family Planning Association
161 Broadway, Sydney 2007 (211 0244)
Menopause Clinic (Royal Hospital for Women)
188 Oxford Street, Paddington 2021 (339 4111)
Women's Medical Centre
8th Floor, Challis House, 10 Martin Place, Sydney 2000 (231 2366)

Women's information services

Women in Crisis Counselling Service
Wayside Chapel, Hughes Street, Kings Cross 2011 (385 6577)
  New South Wales (02 228 7088)
  Victoria (008 135 811 and 03 654 6844)
  South Australia (02 223 1244)
  Queensland (07 229 1580)
  West Australia (09 222 0444)
  Tasmania (002 34 2166)
  Australian Capital Territory (062 75 8108)
  Northern Territory (089 50 3644 and 089 27 7166)
Women's Health Advisory Service
PO Box 1096, Bankstown 2200 (708 4794)

Cancer

Breast Cancer Support Services
NSW Cancer Council, GPO Box 7070, Sydney 2001 (264 8888 from 11am to 2pm)
Cancer Information and Support Society
65 Bay Road, Waverton 2060 (922 2334)

Addiction/dependency/mental illness

Al-Anon
Room 306 Trades Hall, 4 Goulborn Street, Sydney 2000 (264 9255)
Alcohol and Drug Information Service
In Sydney (331 2111) Outside Sydney (008 42 2599 toll free)
Alcoholics Anonymous
127 Edwin St North, Croydon, NSW (02 700 1000)
Alzheimer's Disease and Related Disorders
Wicks Road, North Ryde 2113 (805 0100)
Leichhardt Women's Health Centre
55 Thornley Street, Leichhardt 2040 (560 3011)
Network of Alcohol and Drug Agencies
120 Chalmers St, Surrey Hills 2010 (699 4933)
Samaritans Lifeline
210 Pitt St, Sydney 2000 (264 2222)

Useful addresses in the USA

General

Alzheimer's Disease and Related Disorders
70 E Lake St, Chicago, IL 60601 (800 572 6037 inside IL, 800 621 0379 outside IL)

Consumer's Health and Medical Information Center
PO Box 390, Clearwater, FL 33517
Diabetes Association
1660 Duke St, Alexandria, VA 22314 (800 232 3472)
Epilepsy Foundation
4351 Garden City Drive, Suite 406, Landover, MD 20785 (800 EFA-1000
outside MD)
Multiple Sclerosis Society
205 E 42nd St, New York, NY 10010 (800 624 8236)
National Health Information Center
PO Box 1133, Washington, DC (800 336 4797 outside MD)
National Women's Network
244 7th Street SE, Washington, DC 20003
Spinal Cord Injury Association
149 California St, Newton, MA 02158 (800 969 9629)

Sexual health

AIDS Information Center
Atlanta, Georgia 30333 (800 342-AIDS)
Endometriosis Association
PO Box 92187, Milwaukee, WI 53202 (800 992-ENDO)
National Abortion Federation
900 Pennsylvania Ave SE, Washington, DC 20003 (800 772 9100)
North America Menopause Society
NY Academy of Sciences, 2E 63rd Street, New York, NY 10021
Planned Parenthood Federation
810 7th Avenue, New York, NY 10019 (212 541 7800)
Premenstrual Syndrome Access
PO Box 9326, Madison, WI 53715 (800 237 4666)
Women's Health Advisory Service
PO Box 31000, Phoenix, AZ 85046

Cancer

Breast Cancer Support Program
1757 Ridge Rd, Homewood, IL 60430 (800 221 2141)
Cancer Information Service
Building 31, Room 10A24, 9000 Rockville Pike, Bethesda, MD 20892
(800 4-CANCER)
Papanicolaou Cancer Center
PO Box 016960, Miami, FL 33136 (800 4-CANCER)
USC Cancer Center
1721 Griffin Ave, Room 205, Los Angeles, CA 90031 (1-800 422 6237)

Addiction/dependency/mental illness

Al-Anon Family Group Headquarters
1372 Broadway, New York, NY (800 344 2666)

Office of Drug and Alcohol Programs
Health & Welfare Bldg, Rm 929, 6th & Commonwealth, Harrisburg PA
17120 (800 932 1912 inside PA)
Schizophrenia Association
900 Federal Highway, Boca Raton, FL 33432 (800 847 3802)

Index